Stories of

Love, Hope
and Healing

for All Ages

Joan Zawatzky

First published in Australia in 2017 by Veritax. Victoria, Australia

Website: www.placeofbooks.com

Printing and typeset by BookPOD

ISBN: 978-0-9945532-1-8
eISBN: 978-0-9945532-2-5

For Estelle

Contents

For Older Children & Preteens

STORIES FOR ADULTS AND TEENS
Mindfulness

Embracing Change

Overcoming Obstacles

Growth & Learning

Learning

Healing

Gaining Confidence & Independence

Connections with the Past

A note from the author

Since childhood, stories have enriched my life. Some of my earliest memories are of sitting with my grandmother on her old-fashioned couch listening to her stories while she indulged me with cookies, ice cream, and chocolates. Her stories originated from the *shtetl* (a small town in Eastern Europe*)*, where she was born, and the large city she occasionally visited with wide-eyed excitement. They were powerful and loving stories, full of joy and sadness, and a lesson in the resilience of the human spirit.

My mother's bedtime stories began with "Once upon a time" and opened a magical window to fairies, goblins, giants, lovely maidens and princes. They stirred my imagination and fired my fantasies and dreams. My grandmother and my mother enjoyed telling me stories as much as I enjoyed listening to them. It was our loving connection that enhanced them in my memory.

Sadly, my father's many stories about his escape from the horrors of war-torn Europe, and his years of fighting in North Africa with the Allied Forces were locked away from me. In those times men did not tell war stories to their children. They shared them with other men over a beer.

Later, when I began to write my own stories, I was able to explore ideas, to imagine other people's lives, and visit different places and situations that ordinarily I wouldn't have been able to access.

As a counsellor, I found storytelling a subtle means of helping people trying to cope with troubling issues. Stories allow adults and children to explore their feelings safely, understand how others feel, come to terms with difficult situations, or learn new and positive ways of responding.

After writing and telling many stories, I am convinced that love is one of the most powerful ingredients in stories that heal. Stories inspired by love take us beyond facts. They speak to our hearts and souls.

All the stories in this book are part of me. I have learned so much from writing them, and I am delighted to share my belief in the healing power of love with you. If one story doesn't speak to you loudly enough, try reading another. Listen to your intuition. I hope that you will find the stories enjoyable, that they will tickle your imagination, and inspire you to find your own answers.

Joan Zawatzky

Introduction

Love, hope and healing

Love speaks to our hearts. It is the core of our existence and conveys our deepest emotions of kindness, compassion, gratitude, and empathy. Through it our deepest needs are met.

The strange thing is that everyone has their own interpretation of what love is. For many people love is a feeling, a "liking". But, love is far more than that, and it is not one thing. It occurs on many levels, whether it is romantic love, the care and affection for a child, parents, a pet, or a country. It can be connected to a concept, or be an integral part of religious belief.

Love is an unconditional and passionate commitment to another person, a concept, or activity. The needing and giving of love is the essence of the interdependence we have on one another. It binds us as human beings, keeps families and communities together and gives deeper meaning to our lives.

Love can be uplifting and rewarding, but it can be cruel too, as in the loss of love by rejection, disloyalty, or due to the death or disappearance of a loved one.

Self-love

Self-love is not merely a platitude. Self-love is about knowing that we matter, and that we are worthy of being loved. It is about being kind, caring and considerate to ourselves when we are struggling, sad or unwell. When we value ourselves, and allow ourselves to be who we are, we are able to love others as well. We are open to new ideas and focussed on achieving our own meaning and purpose

Unfortunately, many of us find it difficult to appreciate ourselves. We deny our positive qualities, judge ourselves harshly, and seek approval from others. Self-love is not merely feeling good, being self-absorbed or selfish. It involves accepting our shortcomings as well as our strengths, and having compassion for ourselves when we face life's serious challenges.

For many of us, trying to find a source of self-love can appear fruitless. Early unhappy memories about lack of affection can weigh us down and fill our thoughts with sadness. The idea of unconditional self-love can seem like an impossible fantasy, but if we care about ourselves, we are able to ask for help when we need it, without shame or embarrassment. Caring and appreciating who we are can be a lengthy journey, and we may need help along the way. Sharing ideas and thoughts with supportive, caring people can help us to rediscover love in ourselves.

Healing and Storytelling

When we read a story, we lose ourselves in the lives of others, and without realising it, it touches us.We create our own inner association with our memories, dreams, hopes or experiences. A story can be a powerful echo of the past that affects our present choices, and changes the direction we take. If what we are telling ourselves is negative or unhelpful, or we are not handling a situation well, a story can be an important wake-up call. Stories can help us to develop new ways of thinking about who we are, how we treat ourselves and others.

In ancient cultures healers or shamans were, and still are, storytellers. Elders of the Australian Aboriginal and Native American Indian tribes, as well as other indigenous cultures, have been telling stories about cultural values and traditions to help young people to find their place in a community for thousands of years. Storytelling has been, and still is, included in community rituals as part of healing.

We are all storytellers

We are all storytellers and have our own stories. Storytelling is one of the few universal activities across cultures, past and present. Stories are our basic form of communication and connection. They explain who we are, give meaning to the pattern of our lives and put information into context. Stories are the language of our thoughts and feelings. They are the way we reach out to each other. Our stories entertain, comfort, teach, touch us within, and heal. A crying baby tells the story of his hunger, a tearful child complains to his mother about being bullied at school, partners discuss their day at work, television shows us a new product on the market, and social media spreads stories about occurrences in our community or wider society.

The history of storytelling

Storytelling is the earliest form of spreading knowledge, recording events, maintaining traditions, and cultural and moral values from one generation to another. Even before stories were told orally, people painted their stories on the walls of caves. Ancient Australian Aboriginal rock art is still visible on cave walls. The early Egyptians wrote their stories on papyrus, and carved them in stone. The bible contains some of the earliest stories. Early Mesopotamian, Greek and Roman myths are full of symbolic meaning.

During the Middle Ages, minstrels and troubadours travelled the countryside telling and singing their stories. They were highly respected and in demand, and provided a link to the history of local areas. With the invention of the printing press in the early 1500's books gradually overtook the role of the troubadour storyteller. Though stories remained popular throughout the centuries, the audience no longer sat in a circle around the storyteller to hear them.

Today, storytelling has changed dramatically. Wi-Fi, smart-phones, social media, video, and television play a dominant role in our lives, but stories continue to be an essential way of staying connected, sharing ideas, spreading information, and shaping public opinion. In spite of the numerous technological advances, the simple act of storytelling by an individual to a group of people has been undergoing a revival, and the number of storytelling festivals and associations have increased.

Storytelling has become a significant part of our lives, in families, classrooms, therapy, marketing, and motivational team building, in both sport and business.

Storytelling in the classroom

When a teacher tells a story, a relaxed and intimate atmosphere is created in the classroom. Textbooks, and more recently computers are undoubtedly important necessary tools for learning. When children are listening to a story, they are focussed and involved. They identify with the choices and actions of heroes and heroines which allows them to view situations and their own difficulties from a different perspective.

Storytelling encourages children to read more, it increases their vocabulary, improves their comprehension, memory and listening skills. It inspires children to talk about, and write their own stories.

Stories help to explain concepts and promote discussion. Carefully chosen stories teach children to appreciate individual and cultural differences, or deal with troubling issues, such as bullying, feelings of isolation or lack of confidence. Children who are unmotivated or struggling to grasp abstract ideas find listening to stories an easier and more enjoyable form of learning than textbook learning.

As part of a lesson or to stimulate discussion, teachers can use the stories in this book, or adapt them slightly to highlight a particular issue. Names of characters and places can be altered to suit a particular child or group of children.

Storytelling for parents

Unlike written stories, family stories are free and can be told at any time or place. They provide a bonding experience for parents and children. Though reading stories to children serves an important purpose, telling a child your personal or family story helps to develop a more intense connection. Children will find stories about relatives past and present, or tales about your life intriguing, such as your first day at school, a time you were scared, but overcame your fear, or how you made friends at school.

Stories about your family and culture pass on your values, traditions and heritage. Through stories, children learn where they belong, about acceptable behavior, and actions to avoid. Stories from other cultures help children to understand and respect the differences in lifestyle and traditions of other people as well.

Not all family stories are pleasant, relaxing or have perfect outcomes. For some families, painful or traumatic stories are an important part of their history, and the people they have become. In understanding how problems were resolved and challenges met in the past, children will be inspired to find new ways of solving some of their own difficulties. Telling stories to children is beneficial if told in a positive way, and takes into account the age, emotional and developmental level of children.

Sharing of stories and experiences of the day are a valuable part of the natural communication between parents and their children, and for many, continue well into adult years.

Some suggestions for parents when reading stories to their children:

- Read a story that you enjoy telling as much as your child enjoys listening.

- While a story cannot solve a child's problems, it is a useful tool that can help during a difficult period in your child's life.

- Begin by reading stories that are about topics or situations important to your child, that suit feelings or attitudes at the time. Later, your child may be open to listening to a wider range of stories.

- If your child is bored by a story it may be too simple. A story that causes your child to become restless or distracted may be too complicated, or difficult to understand.

Stories for troubled teenagers

Adolescence is frequently a time of turbulence. Many teenagers feel isolated and vulnerable in our ever changing, complex world. As they begin to assert their independence and find their individual identity, they tend to connect strongly with their peers, and begin to distance themselves from their parents. A teenager struggling to cope with personal issues may be reluctant to turn to a parent for help.

Storytelling is a pleasant, safe and entertaining way for parents and teenagers to communicate. Of course, finding the most appropriate time is important. Relevant stories can be told in a spontaneous and relaxed manner while driving, around a camp fire, during a walk, or while working on a task together.

When teenagers immerse themselves in a story, they identify with the characters and situations. This gives them the opportunity to experiment freely with conflicting values and imagine real life consequences. Stories demonstrate a variety of ways to manage a situation that can translate to real life situations.

Storytelling is an effective way of motivating teenagers in a gentle, constructive way. Some suggestions of helpful stories in this book for young adults are, for example, about bullying at school and online, sexual abuse, leaving home, family relationships, love, gaining self-esteem, overcoming obstacles and dealing with change.

Enjoyment of a story and then sharing ideas and feelings through discussion can deepen existing bonds between parents and teenagers, or regenerate communication.

Storytelling in marketing

Storytelling has become a popular technique used in marketing. A story can set a company or brand apart from its competition by giving it character or personality that draws people to it. The use of power point and bullet lists from an overhead projector in a presentation has its place, but storytelling is a more personal way of imparting information. Facts conveyed are likely to be remembered if they arouse the emotions of empathy, sympathy, anger or amusement.

The brain, science and stories

We have always known intuitively that stories stimulate and inspire us, change the way we think and feel, as well as the way we interact with others.

Recently, neurobiological research using neuroimaging techniques such as MRI scans, have shown that changes in the brain can occur in response to an emotionally charged story. The brain does not make a distinction between a real experience and one we read or hear about. In stories, the brain responds to descriptions of smells and movement, and processes them like an actual encounter. Researchers have found that emotionally compelling stories affect our attitudes and inspire us, allow us to perceive things differently, increase our understanding and empathy for others, and can be motivating.

Research in this fascinating new area is ongoing, and we hope to learn more soon.

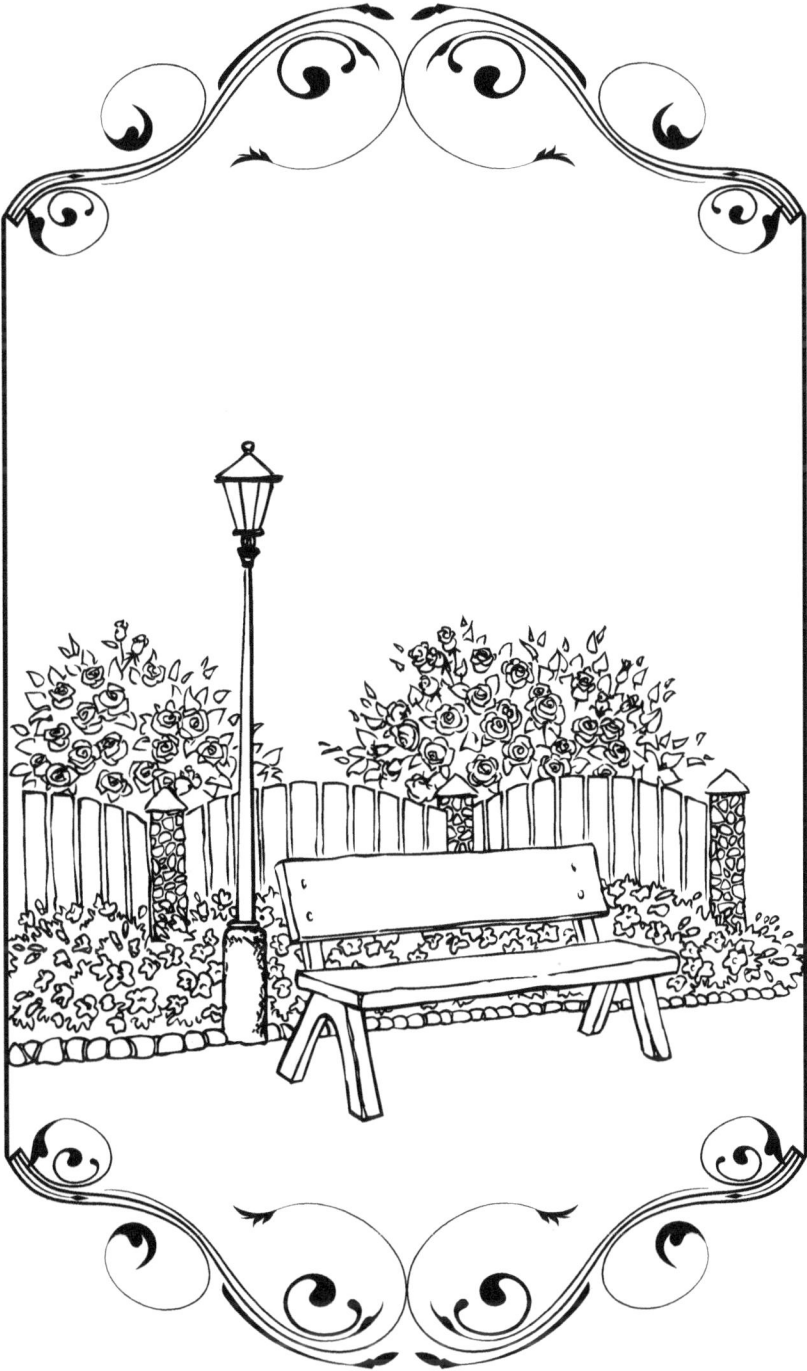

About Families

Family Treasures

The day Sarah and Matthew were married in the small country church, the celebration was tinged with sadness. The couple intended to leave their family and community after the reception. Almost the entire farming community attended the wedding reception as free drinks, food and dancing was an attraction. Sarah's father was not a wealthy man, but that year he had sold his lambs for a good price. He wanted to give the couple a memorable send off. Sarah's sister organised the striped marquee, pink and white flowers to match Sarah's dress, and long tables groaning with food.

Sarah and Matthew led the dancing that continued late into the night. When the band finally packed up their instruments, and the last drinks were served, Sarah's father called his daughter aside. His words pleading her to stay for at least a few more years were on his lips, but he did not speak them. She was his first born and his favourite child, but he had to let her go.

Matthew was ambitious for wealth and success. He was determined to leave the small town for a future in the city. As reluctant as Sarah was to leave her family, she adored Matthew and was prepared to do almost anything to please him.

Sarah's father hugged and kissed his daughter. He then handed her a small red leather box. 'Your mother and I want you and Matthew to have some of our family treasures,' he said. 'When you leave us, our history should be with you, so that you can pass it on to your children.'

The couple's departure from the station was accompanied by good wishes from their families and friends, and a round of tears. Once they had settled in the train for the long journey, Sarah felt in her carry bag for the box her parents had given her.

She ran her fingers over the fine leather. When she opened the box, a familiar photograph of her parents and sister lay against the lid. Beneath the photograph, was a delicate silk scarf with a sprig of blue flowers that had belonged to her grandmother. She stroked the scarf, remembering her grandmother's blue eyes sparkling when she wore it on special occasions. There was a silver teaspoon engraved with a decorative handle that had belonged to her great grandmother. Her mother had used it only for visitors. A tortoiseshell comb inlaid with mother of pearl brought back fond memories of family gatherings, and the fun she once had playing with her cousins. Great aunt Bessie had inherited it from her grandmother and worn it with pride in her long auburn hair. Tucked into one corner of the box was a black velvet pouch containing three gold coins that had belonged to her great grandfather. In the other corner was a small blue case containing a silver brooch in the form of a dove with shimmering wings. The dove's eye was made from a glinting red jewel. It had been a wedding gift to her great-grandmother from her beloved cousin.

Their arrival in the city was exciting, but the couple realised that life there would be more difficult than they had imagined. After searching, they found a small furnished room. It was stark and dreary, but all they could afford. Immediately they both looked for work. Though Matthew had managed a farming co-operative, he was unable to find an administrative job in the city. Sarah had worked as receptionist for a country doctor, but she could not find work either.

'I know how much you wanted to come to the city,' Sarah said, stroking Matthew's hand. 'As much as I love you I wouldn't have agreed to come if I'd known finding a job would be so hard'.

Matthew gave Sarah a kiss. 'Be patient, it will take time to find something that suits us. Meanwhile we might have to take whatever is available.'

Matthew worked as a casual labourer while continuing to look for a more suitable job, but Sarah was still unable to find work. With only Matthew's income their savings dwindled. It was then that Sarah thought of the gold coins. One coin would provide them with food for the month, and possibly go towards paying the rent as well. As reluctant as she was, she took a coin to a pawn broker and returned with a sheaf of money. Now that the red box had been opened, it was as if the seal to the past had been broken.

She was beginning to think that she would never find work, when she noticed an advertisement for a hotel maid. She applied, and started the next morning. While cleaning one of the rooms in the hotel, she met a doctor and his wife, who were staying in the hotel for a few days. When the doctor realised that she had worked as a doctor's receptionist in the country, he offered her a job.

They were just able to scrape by when Matthew came across a carpenter in the city mall who owned a large furniture stall. Matthew's hobby had been carpentry, and over the years he had made almost all his parent's furniture. He knew fine work when he saw it and complimented the carpenter who was flattered. After a friendly chat, the carpenter offered to employ Matthew to help him with office work and basic carpentry.

At last he had a solid job. In his free time he sharpened his skills in carpentry. The couple was able to move into an apartment, and Matthew made all the furniture they needed.

One night, while they were asleep, thieves broke into their apartment. They stole their furniture and most of their possessions. It was a huge loss. Matthew was shattered by the theft of the furniture. Sarah wept over the stolen wedding presents. They were thinking of leaving for home, when Sarah decided to spend the second gold coin on replacing the household items. The sale of the second coin made Sarah feel guilty, but not as guilty as selling the first one.

In the evenings and over the weekends Matthew made furniture, and sold it at markets and fairs. He had learned all he could from his employer and had the beginnings of a small business, but he struggled to buy the wood and other necessary supplies. Without much thought, Sarah sold the last coin to help him on his way.

It was around this time, that Sarah became pregnant with James and left her job. When James was weaned, he refused to take solids. She remembered the decorative spoon in the red box. James was attracted to the spoon's coloured handle and ate from it. From then on, she kept the spoon in the kitchen. Caring for James was exhausting, and she longed to return to work. Fortunately, a neighbour who loved children offered to care for him for a few hours each week. In gratitude, Sarah impulsively gave the kind woman her grandmother's silk scarf.

Eventually, the couple bought a modest house. During the move Sarah tossed the red leather box into a top cupboard. They had all they needed, and with their life more settled, Sarah had another child they called Phyllis.

In the early years after leaving home, she kept in touch with her parents by letter and occasional phone calls. As the months and years passed, she wrote to them less often and their conversations gradually became forced. Her sporadic correspondence with her sister ceased as well. Though she wrote to her parents to inform them about James' birth, they replied that they were too old and sick to travel. She had been away eleven years when her father died suddenly, but she did not attend the funeral. When her mother died four years later, she did not return to the farm either.

Once their children had left home, Matthew and Sarah spent barely any time together. While he carved wooden sculptures in his workroom, she cooked and sewed. Sarah was lonely and often thought of her family and the farm. All she had left were her memories and the few items in the red leather box. She realised then that her father had given her a message about the importance of family ties. The box was her link with the past that she had not valued in her race to establish a new life in the city. After searching through all the cupboards, she eventually found it. Eagerly she opened it, kissed the family photo and gazed at it for a long time. She was relieved to find the silver dove and comb.

She felt guilty about her impulsiveness, but could do nothing about it. Instead of crying about her loss, she valued what was left. She bought an exquisite gold frame for the photograph and placed it on her bedside table. Once she had cleaned the brooch, it shone and its jeweled eye twinkled. Pinning it on her shirt, she admired it in the mirror. She told both her children about the box and about their family. She gave her daughter, who had inherited the family's auburn curly hair, the tortoise-shell comb.

Months later, Sarah visited her parent's graves in the village near the farm where she was raised.

A Mother's Love

Brian was eighteen and had found out recently that he was adopted. He couldn't help being angry that his adoptive parents had not told him earlier that his biological mother was Ellen Laver.

He had been searching for her for the past three years, but so far there was no trace of her. He continued to hope that she was out there, somewhere. He hoped too that she had a good reason for giving him away. If she was still alive, did she ever think about him, he wondered.

After a long wait, the social worker at the government department ushered Brian into her room.

'Good to see you again,' she said with a smile.

He nodded and waited as she looked through her correspondence in a file on her desk.

She looked up. 'We talked about a few places you could write to when we last saw each other. Were there any positive responses to your letters?'

'Not a thing! And I'm beginning to think I'll never find my mother.' His voice was sharp with frustration. 'She must be old by now, or she could be dead.'

The social worker said, 'There's no record of a death certificate.'

He continued speaking fast, 'I understand in a way. Maybe at first my parents, adoptive parents, thought it was best for me not to know about her, but now that they are both in their late fifties with health problems they've changed their minds and decided to tell me the truth. They've always treated me like their loved child. I love them too, but they're not my blood,' he said with a gulp. Since I've known about my mother I feel lost…like I don't belong anywhere. I'm sure I'd feel a lot better if I found her. The way I see it now, I'm nothing.'

'Have your parents told you anything about your mother, Ellen?'

'They explained that they couldn't have children of their own and how badly they wanted me…and I know it's true. They haven't met my mother, and have tried to find her, but had no luck either.'

'This is a very difficult time for you and I don't want to build up your hopes, Brian, but I have some news for you. I was searching through records last week, and came across this.' She handed him a piece of paper with the name of a small town about two hour's drive from the city. 'I'm not sure if it will help. It's an old document, but it's the first solid lead we've had lately about your mother's whereabouts.'

The following weekend, Brian drove through the town's main street, a jumble of cottages, cafés and souvenir shops. He parked under the shade of a tree and entered a quaint cottage café decorated with paintings of the once thriving town before its inhabitants had left for the cities. Inside, an elderly couple, two old women and a few tourists were enjoying afternoon tea. Brian ordered coffee and asked the young man at the counter if any of the people in the café were residents. The man pointed to the two women.

The women remembered Ellen Laver, but said that she no long lived in the town. The older of the two recalled that Ellen had been a beauty, who loved animals and children and fed all the stray cats and dogs in the area. One day she had left suddenly with her animals and moved to a nearby town. No one had seen her since.

During Brian's drive home he wondered about the woman who cared for strays and children, but had given her own child away. There were four other small towns in the vicinity. Brian made enquiries about his mother in them all, but drew a blank. With no further leads, he stopped his search and threw himself into work.

He was a builder, and was constructing an extra room for a couple due to have a baby. After working on the site for a few days, he looked forward to times when the pregnant woman came to check the building's progress, or to bring coffee and biscuits. He was attracted to her warm smile, gentle voice and round shape. In his fantasies, she was the mother he had searched for, and longed to have.

Months later, he received an email from the social worker asking to see him.

'A letter has arrived from Ellen Laver,' the social worker told him. Shocked, he stared at her. 'After all this time! Why now?'

'She'd heard that you had been searching for her. You know how people talk in small towns. She's sick and she wants to see you.'

Angrily he wiped away his tears. 'She's waited all this time to contact me and now that she's sick, she's decided to see me! For my part she can rot like an old piece of timber,' he replied.

'I'll give you her address in case you change your mind,' she said. 'And if you do visit her, please let me know how things turned out.'

Brian wrestled with himself. As much as he longed to meet his mother, he resented her contacting him at this late stage.

A month later he relented and knocked on the door of an old house. A grey haired woman opened the door. 'I'm Flora, Ellen's friend. You must be…?'

'Yes…I'm Brian, her long lost son.'

'Come in, I'll tell Ellen you're here.'

He followed Flora through the narrow hall. As he entered the sitting room he noticed a large photograph of a young woman and baby on the wall. A woman much older than the one in the photo sat in an easy chair. She looked up at him and held out her hands in welcome. He stepped back and stared at her. She was around forty-five, he gauged. Her features were finely chiseled and her green eyes like his, were filled with tears.

At first she was too overcome with emotion to speak. When she managed to talk, it was between tears. 'I can't tell you how blessed I feel to see you again.' She looked at him for some time. 'And you're a fine looking young man too…as I pictured you'd be.'

Brian looked away to control his tears.

'I don't know how I can explain myself to you…make you understand my guilt and torment at letting you go all those years ago.'

Brian didn't reply. He couldn't.

She rocked herself to and fro in the chair trying to calm herself. At last she was able to speak again. 'It's time you heard the real story behind your adoption.'

Brian nodded and took a deep breath, suddenly afraid of what he might hear.

'I've forced myself to stay away from you because I didn't want you to know that all those years ago while you were growing up that I was in jail. Your father and I were part of a gang that robbed a bank. We were all caught and you were born in prison. After a lot of thought, I decided to offer you for adoption to give you the opportunities of a better life. Giving you away was harder than serving my sentence.'

'I had no idea,' he replied.

'Look at the photograph on the opposite wall,' Ellen said. 'In the right hand corner you'll see bars on the window. It was taken just days before the adoption agency took you from me. I've always loved you, but I thought it was wrong to make you bear your parent's shame.'

There was no point then in telling her he would've preferred to know the truth. He would wait for another opportunity to talk about his pain and disappointment.'

'You wrote in your letter that you are sick.'

'Yes, I've had leukemia for a few months. I am taking some new medication and I'm responding to it, so hopefully my health will improve. For some time I've felt that I should tell you the truth about your background. I didn't want to die without you knowing how loved and wanted you were. I've thought about you and imagined how you'd look and what you were doing every day of my life,' she said, as she began to cry again.

'What happened to my father?' Brian asked.

'His name was James. He was killed in prison by a gang member who thought he had hidden more than his share of money from the robbery. It all happened such a long time ago,' she said sadly.

Brian stared at her, too overcome with emotion to reply.

'It must be hard for you to take this all in,' she said.

He nodded.

'I hope you'll understand…and come to see me again in time.'

Brian understood his mother's reason for giving him away, but the hurt in spite of the circumstances, wouldn't leave him.

Two months later, he decided to visit her again, after reminding himself that she was seriously ill. There was so much he wanted to ask her, and it wasn't wise to wait too long.

Her eyes shone with pleasure when he entered the room. This time they were both more at ease and discussed many of the things they had in common. They had the same colour eyes, skin, and hair. Then they discovered that their tastes in music, food and wine were similar too, and that they liked the same books and films.

Ellen responded well to the new medication and was able to leave her home for short periods. Brian visited her often. He took her for coffee or drives in the countryside. They talked a lot, now that they were more comfortable in each other's company. She showed him photographs and told him about her early life, and as much as she knew about his father before they were involved in the robbery. He had many questions about the robbery. She explained how she and his father were out of work after they married. Influenced by her cousin, they agreed to take part in what seemed to be an easy way to improve their lives.

Unfortunately, Ellen's spell of improved health did not last. Almost a year after their first meeting her health declined rapidly. Brian visited her daily at a hospice. When she was almost too weak to talk they said their "goodbyes."

Four months later, Brian visited the social worker for the last time.

'I'm so sorry, Brian. So soon after finding Ellen you lost her.'

'Just when we were getting to know each other, she left me again. But, I have come to terms with her death now. I was lucky to have had the opportunity to share precious moments with her. At least now I know that she loved me…that she gave me away for my benefit.'

'I'm glad you feel like that, Brian. It hasn't been easy.'

'Well, I have some great memories now. I found out more about who I am and where I came from.'

'I'm pleased for you.'

'I became fond of her and I'm sad she has gone, but she couldn't have taken the place of my adoptive parents. They have cared for me since I was a baby, and gave me all the affection I needed. I love them too, and they are my parents.'

Leaving Home

Lorenzo was awakened by the sound of a banging door. Sleepily, he felt for his slippers and went to investigate. In the morning light the house was still. As it was too late to return to bed, he padded into the kitchen to make coffee. It was then that he noticed a letter on the kitchen table addressed to "My Parents". He recognised his son Serge's handwriting and opened it immediately.

Dear Mama and Papa

By the time you read this letter I'll have gone. I can't live at home any longer feeling that you're ashamed to have a son like me. Being gay is who I am, and it is right for me.

You were both born in Italy, where gay people were regarded as second class citizens, scum. In those days, men had to be "macho", marry and have children. Just as well things have changed a lot since the old days. In Italy today, gay men and women are proud of who they are. You've both known I was gay for ages, but you didn't talk to me about it. Think back to what I was like as a child. I wasn't like other boys who played rough and kicked balls. I preferred dolls to trains and machines. Papa, I know you tried hard to interest me in soccer, but I hated it, and was a useless player. Mama, at twelve, you caught me dressing up in your clothes and trying out your make-up and perfume. I did it lots of times and maybe you closed your eyes to it. Surely you realised eventually that I was going through more than "a phase".

Last Christmas, when we were all sitting in the sun relaxing, I delivered my bombshell. There was silence, and neither of you could even look at me. Mama, I know I've destroyed your dreams of my marrying and having kids. A few days after Christmas you suggested I speak to our priest or a counsellor, but I don't see why I should. Perhaps you thought that they could make me straight. Whether you and Papa like it or not, I like who I am and I have no intention of changing.

I know that life as a straight person would be easier in lots of ways, but the easiest way isn't always the best way. If I could live a lie it would be easier for us all. Papa, it was you who taught me that being true to oneself is one of the most important things in life. I love you both, and I'm grateful for the love you have given me, and the sacrifices you made for me. But, I've decided not to stay at school. The bullying is tearing me apart, and I'm not going to put up with it any longer. I have to make a more positive life for myself. I'm sorry to be such a disappointment and a failure.

I'll be staying with friends, but I'll let you know more as soon as I'm settled. I'm seventeen, and able to look after myself. When I find work I hope to move into a more permanent place. Please don't phone and ask me to come home. I have thought about this for a long time and I won't change my mind.

I hope that one day you will accept who I am, and that we will see each again.

Your gay son

Serge

Lorenzo rushed to Serge's bedroom. The room was neater than usual. The bed was covered with a quilt, the cupboards empty. Serge was true to his word, he had gone. 'Lina, Lina wake up!' he shouted, as he waved the letter in his hand. 'Serge has gone…and…he left this letter.' He sat on the edge of their bed, his head in his hands and sobbed.

After Lina had read the letter, her face turned pale, but she did not cry. She had to act, try to do something to bring Serge back home. And there were the younger ones. They adored Serge. What would she tell them?

Lorenzo pushed his breakfast away. He phoned his employer to say he was sick and rushed out of the house. He walked fast along the beach front, until exhausted, he dropped onto the sand. His head throbbed with fury and blame. First his anger was directed at God to have given him a gay son. He moved on to blaming Serge for not trying harder to fight his impulses. Then he blamed Lina for being too soft with Serge.

He stared at the sea seeking answers, but there were none. He loved Serge so much that he ached. He thought about how hard he had tried to be a good father. He had taught Serge about a man's role in the family and the community. It was the only way he knew, but Serge had chosen to ignore, and even reject it all.

As Lorenzo slowly walked home, he recalled Serge's announcement during the family Christmas dinner. It hadn't come as a shock. He turned his anger on himself. Of course he had known for years that Serge wasn't like other boys. Serge was correct, he had refused to accept it. Instead, he had tried to force him to change. He loved Serge and should've accepted him as he was, he told himself shakily. Once home, he went to his study and shut the door.

Over breakfast the next morning, Lina told ten year old Isabella and Jeremy aged five, that Serge was staying with a friend and would be away for a while. They were upset that he had not said "goodbye", but had no idea of the seriousness of their older brother's decision.

Once the children were at school, Lina sat at the kitchen table and wept. Her pain was for her own loss, for the family's loss, and more so for Serge, who had felt so alone and unloved that he had left his family. She was certain that it was her fault. She had failed as a mother, she told herself. If only she had been more understanding when she realised he was gay, and hadn't pretended he would change. Again and again she tried to phone Serge, but he didn't answer her calls or respond to her messages of love. Then she phoned his friends who told her nothing. Desperate she went to her bedroom, not knowing what to do.

Instead of sharing their sadness about Serge, Lina and Lorenzo kept their distance from each other. When they talked, one blamed the other for Serge's absence. A pall of sadness and loss hung over the house. Meals were quiet and eaten quickly instead of being noisy and joyful, as they once were when the family was together. The two younger children missed Serge dreadfully, but eventually they stopped asking when he was returning.

Lorenzo went back to work. He took the train to and from work each day, and for the first time he noticed gay couples. Two young men sitting together whispered to each other. Another two shared a newspaper. Now that he was more aware, he noticed gay people all over the city and elsewhere. He wondered why he had been so blind before.

While the family watched a television newscast one evening, a reporter talked excitedly about the recognition of same-sex marriage in the USA. The celebrations all over the country were shown on the screen. Lina and Lorenzo looked at each other.

Isabella smiled and said, 'Serge will be thrilled.'

'How do you know about Serge?' Lorenzo asked.

'I asked him if he was gay one day, and he said "yes, he was."

'And how do you know about these things?' Lorenzo asked.

'We learned about being gay at school. And there are two great gay boys in my class…we're friends and I trust them with my secrets more than the girls,' she said with a smile.

Later Lorenzo and Lina talked.

'You know Renz, your cousin Antonio is gay, but your brother thinks everyone is blind and can't see it. Antonio is happy in his work as a pastry chef and he has lots of friends. This is not the end of the world for Serge,' Lena said, as she placed her arm around her husband's shoulder. 'He can make a good life for himself.'

'Yes, Antonio is as gay as they come and I do love him. I wish I could've shown that love to Serge,' he said sadly. 'We're both at fault, but I wish I knew what to do.'

Early the next morning Lina woke with an idea. 'Wake up Renz,' she said shaking him. 'I've thought of something we could do.' She didn't wait for him to wake fully, but went on talking. 'We can ask Antonio for dinner and tell him what's happened…maybe he knows already. Serge and Antonio were always close. He'll tell us how Serge is, and maybe he'll be able to help.'

Antonio came for dinner, and after a lengthy conversation he explained that Serge had struggled with his decision to leave school for some time. 'It was constant bullying with no help or support from teachers. When one of the big guys in Serge's class beat him up, Serge was determined to leave.'

'Oh no! We had no idea…and with no one to help him!' Lorenzo said, covering his head with his hands.

Isabella began to cry. 'Poor Serge!'

Antonio hesitated before continuing. 'I know this will be hard for you all. Serge couldn't face going back to school and didn't know how to tell you both how he felt. He knew how badly you both wanted him to complete his studies and maybe go to university…do all the things you weren't able to do, but he couldn't carry on as things were.'

Lorenzo sat silently, wiping away his tears. When he regained his composure, he spoke again. 'You're right Antonio, we both had to leave school early. We had to bring in money for our families to survive. We didn't have a choice, but we wanted the very best for Serge, and our upbringing in Italy made his being gay hard to understand. But, times are different now. We should've realised what he was going through, and given him more support. If only we'd talked more maybe we would've been able to help him.'

'Well…let's hope for change in the future,' Antonio said.

Lina rubbed her hands worriedly. 'I hope he's alright…has enough food and is comfortable.'

'I know where Serge is staying, but he asked me to keep it secret. Try not to worry. He's settled and he'll be fine.'

Lina nodded.

At the door Antonio gave them all hugs. 'I'd like to see you all together and happy again, so I'll tell him how much he is loved. Try not to worry. Give him some time. I'm pretty certain that you'll both be able to tell Serge yourselves how much you care about him. Then it's up to him to decide if he wants to come home.'

Isabella clutched Antonio's hand to stop him leaving. 'I miss Serge so much. I'm so sad that he felt we didn't understand him. I wish I could give him a big hug… now!'

Jeremy spoke for the first time. 'He's my big brother and I miss him lots and lots.

'If I write him a letter will you give it to him, Antonio?' Isabella asked.

Jeremy interrupted. 'I want to write too.'

'Of course I'll give him your letters,' Antonio said, as he stepped back into the house. 'I'll wait for you to write the letters, and give them to him as soon as I can.'

Lina clapped her hands. 'That's a wonderful idea. We can write to him too and tell him how much we love him…that we are so sorry that we let him down…and that we hope he forgives us. We can ask him if he would agree to talk about it. What do you think Renz?'

'A very good idea…you need to talk,' Antonio said.

Antonio gave Serge the letters and his family's messages of love. Overcome by the outpouring of love, Serge agreed to meet his parents at a café rather than at their home. After a slow start, they talked openly. Tears and hugs followed his parent's apologies.

'I'm so pleased we met today. We needed to talk. I love you and didn't mean to hurt you like I did, but I couldn't…'

'No need to say anything more about it Serge. We understand and accept your choices…though it was hard for us at first. We're old fashioned people, but we love you and want you to be happy whatever you chose to do,' Lorenzo said.

Serge gave his parents another hug.

'Of course we want you to come back home, and we hope you do, but that's for you to decide,' Lina said, as she took Serge's hand.

'I know you'll both be upset, and Isabella and Jeremy too, but at the moment I need my independence and to sort myself out away from home.'

Lorenzo looked down to hide his distress. 'I'm disappointed, but I left home when I was a little younger than you, so I understand.'

Lina interrupted. 'Even if you aren't living at home, we hope to see you for dinners and chats over coffee…and Isabella and Jeremy want to see you so much.'

'I'll be there Mama! There's nothing to beat your *Osso Bucco* and *Lasagna*.'

What Children Know

Olivia, Peter and their daughter Ella, aged five, returned from their holiday refreshed.

'It was a lovely holiday,' Ella said wistfully, as she closed her eyes, remembering.

'Yes it was, my darling,' Olivia said. 'It was you who asked if we could go back to the mountains and lakes again. How did you know that we all needed a holiday?'

Ella shrugged. Her blue eyes turned misty. 'There was too much shouting at home and it made me very sad. I remembered how much a holiday helped last year.'

Olivia thought of the picture of the family Ella had drawn a few days before they went away. It depicted the three of them standing stiff and disconnected. The small girl in the drawing held her doll and was crying.

'I'm happy now,' Ella said.

'I'm so glad darling...and you drew such a happy loving picture of us all when we came home,' Olivia said, pointing to a drawing on the fridge door.

Ella smiled.

'You know a lot for your age,' Olivia said and gave Ella a kiss.

That weekend they visited Ella's grandmother, Roseanne, for afternoon tea. There were hugs and kisses all round. Then they sat down to the chocolate cake, scones and sandwiches Roseanne had made to welcome them home.

'This is delicious,' Olivia said to her mother, as she licked cream and jam from her fingers. 'Thank you for going to all this trouble for us.'

When Roseanne asked about the holiday, Peter said, 'It was great… comfortable accommodation and wonderful scenery. We couldn't ask for more. We had lots of time together…just what we needed.'

When Roseanne went into the kitchen to boil more water, Ella followed her. She delved into her pocket and produced a folded piece of paper. 'I made this for you Gran. I missed you lots on holiday,' she said, as she placed her drawing on the table. It portrayed a girl and her doll surrounded by creatures with wings. All had smiles and were in light, bright colours.

'It's beautiful. It's you and your fairies. Thank you Ella my love.'

Ella stood quietly for a moment, and then looked around. 'Mum and dad won't be able to hear us in the kitchen will they?'

'They're too busy talking,' her grandmother replied with a laugh.

'I have something to tell you Gran, and I know that they won't believe me.'

'I'll believe you.'

'On holiday I saw fairies in the trees. When I closed my eyes very tight they lifted me up into the sky so that I could fly with them.'

'You're very lucky. When I was your age I saw fairies too,' Roseanne said, and hugged her granddaughter. 'They visited me when I lonely and made me happy again.'

'Yes, my fairies come to visit me when I am lonely or sad too. I saw them lots of times before we went away when Mum and Dad were busy and didn't have time to be with me. One of the fairies, Belinda is special and I love her.'

'Tell me about Belinda.'

'She's pretty with blonde hair, green eyes and she has gold wings. Her voice is sweet and kind, and she tells me lots of secrets.'

'Yes, secrets are the best part,' Roseanne said.

Later Peter was talking when Ella interrupted him. 'Dad, please tell Gran what happened to Mum during the holiday.'

'Well, it's quite a story,' Peter said, as put his cup down and leaned back. 'One morning we left Ella at the hotel with a minder while the two of us went for a long walk. It had been raining overnight and the ground was soggy. Unfortunately Olivia slipped and tumbled. She was in such pain that for a moment I thought she had broken her leg. But, we realised she had probably sprained her ankle. I tore a strip of material from my shirtsleeve and wet it in the nearby stream. After I'd bandaged her ankle we rested for a while. By then, some of the swelling and pain had eased. She was able to hobble back to the hotel with the aid of a branch. After resting, she could walk again.'

'Ella, now it's your turn to tell Gran your part of the story,' Olivia said with an encouraging smile.

'I had a horrible feeling right here…and here.' Ella pointed to her stomach and forehead. 'I knew something was wrong with mum. I told the lady looking after me, but she told me not to worry, and that nothing bad would happen. I didn't believe her, so I asked the fairies to keep her safe and bring her home…and they did.'

Olivia gathered Ella in her arms and kissed her. 'My darling Ella, we love you so much!'

Peter threw his hands up. 'What do you make of that, it's spooky!'

'I'm so pleased it ended well and that you all enjoyed the rest of the time in spite of your nasty experience,' Roseanne said.

They had another slice of cake, and then Peter clapped his hands together to make an announcement. 'We haven't told you our special news,' he said, as he put his arm around Ella.

'You will have a tiny brother or sister soon, my darling.' Olivia said to Ella.

Ella smiled broadly. 'I knew all the time,' she replied with a smile. 'The fairies told me.' She produced another crumpled drawing from her pocket and held it up. She had drawn herself, her doll and the fairies with smiles. A pram with a baby inside it stood next to her mother.

'I give up!' Peter said looking flabbergasted. 'She couldn't have known. We didn't say a word about it to her, or to anyone else.'

'How wonderful, another grandchild!' Roseanne said and kissed Peter and Olivia.

'You're a very special sensitive little girl. Soon you'll have a baby brother or sister to play with as well as your doll,' Olivia said.

'You'll always be our much loved first child, Ella...so don't ever forget how much we love you, Peter said. 'The new baby will need looking after. I'm going to take on extra staff so that I can help out, and there will be more time for us to be together as a family.'

'I'm going to need your help too,' Olivia said to Ella.

'The fairies told me that I'm going to be very happy. They said that they are going on their holiday...so I won't see them anymore.' Ella said with a sigh. 'I will miss them, especially Belinda, but they need a holiday too.'

A Family Learns to Love

Joseph clenched his fist in frustration. *Why is God punishing me? What have I done to deserve this?* He was a tall, imposing Jewish man, who looked older than his fifty-two years. He owned a clothing shop that had belonged to his father. The business had been successful until a new freeway was built. The freeway cut travelling time for motorists by redirecting traffic from the small town where Joseph and others had their businesses. The once thriving shops stood empty of customers as people were unwilling to travel through a choked intersection to reach them. As profits from the shop dropped alarmingly, Joseph worried about his family's future. He didn't tell his wife Estelle or his children how worried he was, but hung on, reluctant to close down.

Daniel, Joseph and Estelle's sixteen year old son, played the clarinet and was set on studying music.

Joseph tried to steer his son towards a career in accountancy or law instead. 'At least you'll have a stable profession and be able to feed a family one day,' he said. 'After all, you can play your clarinet as much as you like over the weekend.'

Daniel refused to even discuss his father's suggestion, and the atmosphere between the two grew tense.

The stress of his business troubles plus the lack of communication with his son made Joseph stressed. He knew that he had to break through the wall between himself and Daniel, but it seemed too hard and he tried to ignore it.

One night, a friend of Daniel's arrived at the house. Joseph usually sent all Daniel's friends straight up the stairs to his son's room, but this young man was a little older than the others and had not been to the house before. Joseph knocked on Daniel's bedroom door to tell him he had a visitor. As the door of his son's bedroom opened, he sniffed a pungent odour. Marijuana. Joseph had smelled it on Daniel's clothing and hair recently, and in his room. He closed his son's door quickly and said nothing.

Daniel's marijuana smoking was another matter Joseph refused to face. He turned to his past for comfort instead. He focused on his pleasant memories of his mother and sister. Losing himself in daydreams, he chose to push away memories of the hard times his immigrant parents endured, the family's poverty and the bullying he had experienced at school.

He longed to be in his childhood home. When his yearning became overwhelming, he drove to the suburb where he had grown up and searched for his childhood home. The houses in the streets looked nothing like he remembered them. Initially, he was stunned that the semi-detached cottage, once his home, was now painted pale apricot and its ornate gable, which he'd admired so much as a child, was dark green. After looking at the house for a while, he admitted to himself that the modern changes made the house more attractive. It's time to stop living in the past, he told himself.

On Friday nights, Joseph usually attended synagogue alone to celebrate the start of the Sabbath. Hoping to repair the rift between them, one Friday Daniel agreed to accompany his father. Though they sat side by side, they barely talked to each other.

Joseph continued to use his father's torn prayer book. It gave him a sense of comfort and connection with the past. With the old book in his hand, Joseph prayed for guidance. The cantor's singing and the mumble of prayers in the background led him to a deep place within, and he asked himself why his son was smoking marijuana. He thought about the age gap between them, and acknowledged that there was much he did not understand about his son. *Daniel is a talented musician. He has won awards at school and at eisteddfods for his clarinet playing. Am I wrong to try to steer him away from a career in music towards steadiness and practicality? All I've achieved for my efforts is resentment.*

As Joseph recited the ancient prayers that were a part of his life, he became less aware of sounds or movements around him, but he was aware that he and Daniel were surrounded by a cocoon of light. He felt so close to Daniel right then. They were one, blended into a flickering, pulsating glow. Soon the clatter of the congregation standing interrupted his peace. The service was over.

While they walked home, the silence between them continued. As they neared the house Daniel talked at last. 'Dad, did you experience a weird sensation ... a warmth…a light?'

'Yes, indeed. The warmth of the Sabbath is a gift,' Joseph answered clumsily, putting his arm around his son.

'I think you're right, Dad,' Daniel replied.

Joseph opened the gate and looked at his son. 'We have a lot to talk about, Dan.'

'Yeah, I guess we do.'

'I don't know if you realise how much I love you and how important you are to me. I've been at fault…ignored your talent…been too self-absorbed,' Joseph said, as they walked into the house together.

Daniel nodded.

Joseph put his hand on his son's arm. 'Dan, I'm worried about you smoking marijuana, but I haven't said a word to your mother. It would upset her too much.'

'I don't smoke much. It helps me to unwind when I'm under pressure at school, and it allows me to get off to sleep at night. Anyway it's no big deal. All the kids in my class smoke it.'

The following week they talked more easily as they walked to synagogue again.

'Dad, I'm worried about you too. I can see you're not yourself. You seem uptight and look tired most days.'

'I know, I'm not feeling right. I'm sorry, I should have told you that I'm extremely worried about what's going to happen with the shop. I haven't done anything about it, hoping things might improve.'

They continued walking slowly. Both were deep in thought.

Joseph turned to Daniel. 'You're not yourself either, Dan. What's upsetting you?'

'My music dad. I'm crazy about it, especially the clarinet, and you've been against it. I think I've got the talent and that's what I want to do…to make it my career.'

'I'm sorry, Dan. I should've known how important it is to you and not tried to push you in another direction. All I wanted was the very best for you.' His voice faded.

'Yeah well let's forget it. The trouble is that I can't even play right now, I've been feeling down lately.'

'When did it start?' Joseph asked, looking worried.

'There's been a lot of pressure at school. The stuff we were learning hasn't made much sense to me. I haven't been coping well, so I increased the amount of marijuana I was smoking to feel better, but it hasn't worked.'

Joseph sighed as they walked up the synagogue steps, 'I had no idea you were having trouble at school and feeling like that. You should've told us.'

'Yeah, we're both under stress and I guess we both should've talked about it…been more open,' Daniel said, as they found their usual seat.

After dinner, Joseph and Estelle talked well into the night. This time Joseph told his wife the truth about himself, the shop and Daniel.

'I'm so relieved you've told me what the trouble is…at last,' Estelle said, as she wiped away a few tears. 'I saw you looking tired and sick and Dan looking sad, not playing his clarinet, and not eating much. I've been terribly worried. Whenever I tried to find out from either of you what the problem was, I couldn't get answers.'

'Daniel and I must be more alike than I thought,' Joseph said with a half-smile.

'At least we are talking to each other now and we can help each other,' Estelle said with an exasperated sigh. 'We need some help, Joseph. The problem with the shop won't go away on its own. Maybe you can talk to Jack next week. He's an excellent accountant and a good friend, and he will give you the advice you need.'

Joseph gave his wife a kiss. 'You're right as always, Estelle. I have some important decisions to make. I'll go and see Jack and our solicitor too. There are some tricky issues involved.'

Joseph told Dan about his discussion with his mother.

'Doing something about it will help dad, I'm sure.' Dan said as he was about to leave for school.

'Just a moment Dan,' Estelle said, putting her hand out to stop him. 'You need to talk to someone who can help you too. Marijuana could become a dangerous addiction. And then there are your problems at school. If it's alright with you, I'll phone our doctor and ask for a referral to a young counsellor.'

'I'd like to talk to someone, but what if I don't trust him or her?'

'We'll keep trying until we find the right person, someone you feel comfortable with.'

Dan nodded. 'Thanks Mum.'

'Well then, let's stick to our plan. I'm sure things will start to fall into place.' Estelle said.

Joseph looked at Dan and then at Estelle. 'I think you've sorted us out, Estelle.'

Johnno and his Mother

Johnno was seven when his father left his family early one morning, and was not seen or heard of again. Johnno and his mother, Sonia, moved from their comfortable suburban house to number 4B at the Bellevue, a once majestic apartment block overlooking the sea, built in the 1920's.

By the time he was thirteen, Johnno was smaller than most of his friends, but he compensated for his size by building up his lean torso at the gym. The lost, forgotten look about him with dark spikes of hair falling untidily on his forehead, and his grey eyes often absorbed in daydreams, appealed to girls.

He went to his classmate's parties and played sport, but avoided close friendships. Though he appeared carefree, he felt different from others of the same age. Since his father's disappearance he was distrustful of others. Some of his classmates had divorced or separated parents, but they all had fathers. In spite of his mother Sonia's attempts to make up for his lack of a father, her dark moods and sharp, quick temper turned him away from her. Since a recent promotion at work, stress had raised her voice several decibels. All the photographs he had seen of her smiling happily belonged to the past.

Johnno barely talked to his mother. To survive living with the 'Witch', as he called her in moments of desperation, he blocked her out of his life so effectively, that he could be near her without being aware of her presence. In his bedroom, he turned his music up, or wore headphones so that her voice couldn't reach him.

After work, Sonia was usually cooking and had no idea that when Johnno disappeared, as he often did, that he took the flight of steps up the fire escape to the area the landlord called the roof garden. Actually, it was a concrete slab used mainly for storing packing cases and junk. In the farthest corner of the slab, Johnno had built a solid hutch for his eight, neutered rabbits and secured it from theft with a complex series of locks. He insulated the hutch against the elements and made it comfortable with soil from the downstairs garden. The two angoras, Nelson and Celeste were large and white, while Reginald, Myrtle, Cynthia, Basil, Daphne and Freddy were dappled, dwarf rabbits. He loved each one.

Johnno changed the soil in the hutch daily and fed his rabbits fresh salad scraps, begged from the fruit shop on the corner. The special food from the pet shop to keep their coats shiny gobbled up the extra money he earned from a newspaper round. The longhaired angoras had to be combed daily and they all needed exercise. He made a run for them, and took them out one at time. Used to his attention and his loving strokes, they sat at his feet waiting until he took notice of them.

Only one other person knew about the rabbits, Harry Ronsky from apartment 6C. He was a fit bachelor, with an almost bald head except for a few grey-brown strands he drew across the top of his head, in the pretense of still having some hair. Harry went upstairs each morning to breathe in the sea air while exercising. The idea of rabbits as pets intrigued him. In his youth in Romania, he had shot them in the mountains. His mother had prepared them to make a delicious stew, and the memory lingered.

One afternoon, Johnno raced up the steps as usual to find Celeste lying on her side hardly moving. Alarmed, he placed her under his jumper for warmth, and took her to the vet. Due to his youth and his many rabbits, he had a special arrangement with the vet and paid him half the usual fee.

'Don't worry, it's only an infection. I'll give her an antibiotic shot, but try to keep her warm and she'll recover,' the vet said kindly.

Before entering the apartment, Johnno checked the garage. The Witch wasn't home yet. He carried the sick animal into his bedroom and made her comfortable on his chair. He hadn't brought one of the rabbits inside before, and quite liked the idea. A cardboard box he found served as a litter box. Her water and food went on plates from the kitchen.

After his evening meal, he returned to his room. While Celeste was asleep on the chair, he listened to music until he felt sleepy. At daybreak, he was awakened by movement. Celeste must have been feeling better and had jumped onto his bed. Her cold, quivering nose told him that she had overcome the infection. Unfortunately, she had left some brown traces of her progress on the bed cover.

'Time for you to go back to your friends upstairs,' he said to the rabbit, as he pulled on his tee shirt. After depositing Celeste in the hutch, he attempted to clean the evidence of her visit. He did the best he could, dressed, swallowed a bowl of cornflakes and rushed out of the door late for school.

As usual before work, Sonia tidied the apartment. In Johnno's room she opened the windows and smoothed down his bed. It was then, that she noticed the brown patches on his bed. At first she wondered if he was ill, but his enormous appetite at breakfast made her discount that theory. Unable to fathom the reason for the stains, she decided to keep a closer eye on her son. She checked his bed for telltale signs, but there were none.

When Sonia noticed him climbing the outdoor staircase to the roof, she followed him as he made for what seemed to her to be a wooden structure. As she crept closer she saw a large animal hutch. Being far sighted, she mistook the small creature he was holding for a rat and gave a terrified yell.

Johnno swung round angrily, 'Can't you bloody leave me alone!'

Ignoring him, Sonia moved closer. 'Ah, so you're keeping rabbits,' she said in a gentle voice. 'What beautiful angoras and lovely dwarfs. Now I understand the mess on your bed cover,' she said smiling.

'Celeste was sick.' He pointed to the plump angora. 'The vet said she needed warmth, so I brought her inside overnight.'

'Is she better,' she asked, looking concerned.

'Ye…es.' He looked at her quizzically, wondering why she was interested.

'Let me hold that darling little brown and beige one in the corner. He's so cute.'

Surprised, Johnno passed Freddy to her. She made soft, clucking noises to the rabbit as she stroked it.

Could the Witch love animals as he did?

Sonia asked the names of all the rabbits and about their food. She told him about a rabbit she had owned as a child and about her other pets. It was the longest and most pleasant conversation between mother and son for ages. Once they were back inside the apartment conversation did not flow as easily. They talked occasionally, but always about the rabbits. Sonia enquired after their health, or if he had enough food for them. Johnno answered tersely.

He noticed that on days his mother worked an afternoon shift, the keys to the hutch were not in the place that he had left them. Uneaten carrot tops and remains of greens he had not fed his pets became regular signs that his mother had paid them a visit. The rabbits were thriving and their coats were even glossier than before.

As hard as Johnno tried, he could no longer block his mother out of his thoughts. Since their meeting on the roof, she had become a person again. She seemed calmer, and though still a tyrant for neatness, even smiled occasionally.

One summer morning, Johnno woke early and with time to spare before school, paid the rabbits a visit. He was shocked to find his mother and Harry Ronsky exercising together on the roof. He watched them from behind a pile of junk. Their exercise consisting of a few bends and jumps was obviously an excuse to meet. He had not seen his mother in a flirtatious mode before and held his hand over his mouth to stop his laughter. Other than on photographs, he had never seen his mother so happy.

Several months later, Sonia decided to leave her stressful job and work closer to home. Apart from minor disagreements, Johnno and his mother talked often. Sonia and Harry Ronsky spent a lot more time together. Harry enjoyed cooking and regularly invited Sonia and Johnno for lunch on Sundays. Johnno looked forward to the rich, tasty food that Harry said was made according to Harry's Romanian mother's recipes. Though Johnno thought Harry a bit strange, he enjoyed his company. It didn't take long for them to discover that they both liked cycling and watching football, though they followed different teams. Johnno joined Harry in his early evening rides along the beach cycling path. On Saturdays the two sat in front of the television together supporting their football teams, and eating Harry's home baked pies.

The change in Johnno was noticed by his class mates. He looked happier, made jokes and was fun to be with. Proudly he told them about his rabbits, and showed them photos and videos. After school he invited Danny, an animal lover, to see his rabbits. Once Danny had left, Johnno sat in front of the hutch with Reginald on his lap. 'Things are changing around here, and it seems for the best,' he said to the rabbit, stroking its floppy ears.

Payback Time

I am in my car trying to find the courage to knock on the door of the house across the road. As I view the large home and well-kept garden, a mixture of resentment and hurt flows through me. My father lives there with his second wife and two young children, my half brother and sister. It is eleven years since I have seen him, or had any contact with him. He left soon after mum died. I was eight then, and my brother Leo was five. We knew it was irresponsible and uncaring of him to leave us, but we were pleased to see him go.

Mum was sick and in hospital a lot of the time. She couldn't care for me and Leo, so we moved in with my grandparents. They had a small apartment near the city. It was cramped with the four of us, but we were loved and cared for.

Mum died soon after we had moved. She had been in pain most of the time in spite of the powerful medications. I kept quiet about my troubles with my father when I was with her, as I knew she would be upset. Mum was warm and gentle, and I will always miss her.

I have put off this visit to my father many times. If I hadn't promised Jeremy, my counsellor, that I'd confront my father, I'd drive away. There is a lot I have to say to him about the way he abused me as a young child. He's going to try to wriggle out of admitting it. He is the sort of man who doesn't admit he's wrong or apologise. I know he will be shocked when I tell him that I have charged him with sexually assaulting me. I am sure he hasn't thought I'd ever have the guts to do it, but thanks to Jeremy, I have been to the police.

To calm my nervousness, I take a few deep breaths and try to find the courage to leave the car, to walk to the house. I have rehearsed what I'm going to say to him over and over. To satisfy myself, I repeat it one last time.

'Look into my eyes and you'll know what you've done, how you've ruined my life. Thank goodness Leo was young enough to escape the treatment you handed out to me. You didn't abuse him, but you gave him no affection. All these years, I've wondered what being our father meant to you, especially now that you have two other children. You didn't care for us, or show us any love. You did harm instead. Maybe you don't have feelings. Many times I heard you say to me that I "wallowed in emotions like a woman." Well, I can tell you what "father" means to me. Fear! When I was four years old I learned not to trust you, or other adults. You brought me cuddly toys - bunnies and dogs, and then took them away if I did something you thought was wrong. But, what did I do? "No questions!" I didn't dare ask, or you would lash out at me with your barbed tongue, and your belt.

Your gifts of sweet, smooth chocolate, "something special for you, my special boy", became associated with pain and fear. By the time I was seven, I lay in bed on edge, listening for your late night footsteps, doors creaking and knobs turning, hoping that alcohol would stop you. Most times it didn't. I pretended to be asleep. Pretended not to notice the bed covers being pulled back, your putrid smell and the jar of your weight, as you eased yourself into my bed. It's strange how the hurt part of me quickly learned not to feel the pain. In my mind, I escaped to the safety of my tree house, where you couldn't reach me. As hard as I tried not to remember, each morning I woke with feelings of disgust and humiliation.

When you left us early that morning, believing no one would hear you go, I danced in the dawn light. At last we were free of you.

I knew exactly what I wanted to say to my father and I would not falter. I wasn't interested in his response. I did not want to know about his problems, or about his troubled youth. What mattered to me was that at last I would confront my father about the way he had abused me as a child.

I opened the car door, crossed the road and walked to his house with confident steps. It was payback time.

Easter Celebrations

Manos loved his wife Alena, but he had a stormy relationship with her brother, Steve. A recent argument between the two men led to them screaming abuse at each other. If Alena hadn't stopped them, they could've reached the punching stage.

Alena's parents were upset by the bad feeling. They worried that family closeness would disintegrate. With Easter celebrations approaching, they nagged Alena to ensure that there would be harmony in the family. Alena tried to ease her parents' concerns, as they talked of little else.

That year, Easter coincided with Alena and Manos' grandchild, Sophie's fourth birthday, a reason for a double celebration. Alena wanted a party with friends and family, but Manos wasn't at all enthusiastic. When Alena became insistent, Manos finally agreed.

'Okay, we'll have a birthday party for Sophie and our usual Easter celebration with all the trimmings. The family and our friends will come, but I'm not happy about inviting Steve and Helen.'

Alena began to cry. 'I'm always the one in the middle. What am I going to tell my parents?'

'I'll have to think about it,' Manos said storming off.

Whenever Manos thought about celebrating with Steve as a guest he became angry. He could not find a way to accept his brother-in-law into his home, let alone his heart.

Alena tried to tell Manos that Easter was a time for forgiveness, but he muttered to himself, ignored her and walked away. She understood Manos' hurt feelings, but what was she to do.

Three weeks before Easter, Manos had a dream he called "a strange and spectacular MGM masterpiece." The next morning he described the dream to Alena in detail.

Our darling Sophie looked pretty in pink. She was singing, and three small cherubs hovered around her. A long table on the patio was laden with traditional food - red eggs, Easter cookies, honey balls, plaited breads, dips, dolmades, fish, and smoked salmon. The aroma of lamb grilling on a spit was everywhere. Large, empty, silver platters waited for slices of the tender meat.

The dream moved on to the arrival of the guests who brought gifts and loving Easter blessings. Then the focus was on Steve and Helen, who arrived last. I felt uncomfortable seeing them, but I welcomed them. Helen brought even more gifts than the others. Steve mumbled that he had "some humble pie to offer." The cherubs twittered amongst themselves and hid their plump faces behind their hands.

Between sips of wine and beer, the young men in their shirtsleeves told jokes, while they kept an eye on a lamb roasting on the spit. Then the food table developed a surreal glow as everyone tucked in, demolishing the mountain of food. The cherubs giggled and pranced as they watched people eating.

Every now and again, one of the cherubs slipped down to the table to grab a handful of cookies and honey balls, and distributed them amongst the others. While the two smaller cherubs were eating, the largest cherub, who was still hungry, flew down to the table to snatch extra food. The other two laughed and whispered to each other. Immediately the large cherub dropped the food and apologised for his greed. Instead of recriminations, he received kisses on both cheeks.

After the meal, the guests played games. Then there was coffee with baklava, and trifle laced with sherry. Everyone patted their tummies and complained of having eaten too much, but there was still room for chocolates.

While the others were enjoying themselves, Steve sat alone. I felt bad for him. I didn't like the idea of any guest in my home feeling that way. The dream lens shifted to the living room, where we all formed a circle and held hands as we began to dance. Above the cherubs were dancing too. This is the best part of the dream. I approached Steve and asked him to join me in the centre of the circle. The two of us danced faster and faster healing our differences, while above us cherubs danced too. The noise of the dancing became so loud that I woke.

Manos put his arm around his wife's shoulder. 'The dream was so real that it took me a while to realise it was morning and I was still in bed.'

Alena sighed. 'What a beautiful dream!'

'It certainly was.'

'Angels that eat, only happen in dreams,' she said with a grin. 'You must've had our Easter party and Steve on your mind.'

He nodded. 'The little cherubs brought me a message, a way of sorting things out and I'm grateful.'

'Oh?'

'I was being inflexible. Steve is a few years younger than me, and he has new ideas. I don't always agree with him, but I need to be more tolerant…and he needs to respect my feelings too.'

'Yes, that's true. You each have a right to your views,' Alena said.

'We are family and Easter is not the time for grudges. I will visit him and try to resolve the bad feeling between us. I hope that he, Helen and the family will join us for the celebration.' Manos said.

Alena gave Manos a kiss.

Loving Couples

Partners

David sat on one end of the drab couch and Marilyn on the other. The television bleated senseless messages as the motel's neon sign flashed endlessly. They had barely spoken to each other for days, and if not for their two young children, they would've gone their separate ways. In a last grab to rescue their marriage, Marilyn had suggested leaving their children with her mother, so that they could spend a week away together. She had hoped that the long drive and overnight stay at a motel on their way to a luxurious sea side villa would provide an opportunity to talk. Not wanting to be the one to pronounce the death of their marriage, David agreed.

Through the thin motel wall, they heard each painful word of a row between a couple in the room next door. A woman's choked voice pleaded, 'Tell, tell me that you love me.' There was a cutting silence and then, 'You won't leave me, will you?'

The man didn't reply, but cleared his throat and the sound reverberated through the walls.

'Get rid of her…please,' the woman begged.

'I don't know,' the man said haltingly. 'I need time…to sort myself out.'

There were sounds of sobbing.

'I've loved you so much…and for so long. Why? What made you betray me like this?' The woman thumped the wall as she spoke. 'If you go back to her, I'm gone, and I'll take Jude with me.'

'Stop piling on the pressure. I need some space…and don't you dare make threats about taking Jude!'

As the argument escalated, David and Marilyn looked down, unable to face each other. Hearing their own situation played out in the next room shook them both. David's dark head was bent, his lips trembled. A surge of resentment raced through him, as he thought of Marilyn's lack of interest in him after Heidi, their second child, was born. Both children had consumed all Marilyn's time and affection. Guiltily he thought of Gina, the woman he had met at a work seminar. She was attractive and good company. Most of all she listened to him. Ending their affair meant having to stop seeing her, and he wasn't sure if that's what he wanted to do.

Marilyn shielded her teary eyes with her hand. She recalled how she had stood by David in the early days while he developed his business, doing without, so that he, Heidi and Gavin could have occasional treats. Then after many long, lonely evenings waiting for him to come home, she had discovered that he was with Gina.

In the early morning, the biting cold hung between them, as they resumed their car journey in silence. Locked in their misery, they did not notice the rising sun caressing the mountain peaks, the crystal dew drops, or the wild, noisy rush of birds. The sunlight did not last and dark clouds claimed the sky with pelting rain.

Suddenly, an oncoming truck swerved towards them on the slippery road. David turned the wheel wildly to avoid it, but it was too late. The last thing he heard was Marilyn's scream, and a shuddering bang.

When a passing motorist stopped, he found David's body slumped over the steering wheel. Marilyn was thrown out of the car onto the road. He called an ambulance, and they were raced to the local hospital. Fortunately, both survived the collision, but were unconscious. The truck driver walked away from the accident though his truck was badly damaged.

As Marilyn struggled to wake in their shared hospital room, she slipped back to loving times with David. They were strolling on a beach hand in hand after a night of passion. Then they walked down the aisle on their wedding day, all hope, smiles, white tulle and flowers. He gripped her hand, and glanced at her admiringly. She felt him stroking her head to ease her pain, as she gave birth to Heidi.

Loud voices and the smell of antiseptic interrupted her memories as she began to surface in the white room. Apart from scratches and bruises, she was unhurt. The doctors said that all she needed was rest.

David was more seriously injured and he remained unconscious for longer. While he struggled to wake, he recalled their love making on the rug in front of the fire, and tenderly holding each other afterwards. Then she was in the kitchen baking a layered chocolate cake especially for him, his favourite since childhood. The scene changed, as he saw her in her navy suit, cool and efficient, helping him to run the office. The images of them both and the children kept changing.

He heard Marilyn calling his name. Though the past was seductive her voice was insistent. When he opened his eyes, he first saw nurses and a doctor in a white coat. When he looked around he saw Marilyn in the bed next to him, and heard the soft sounds of her praying.

Their hands moved across the beds, over the starched sheets towards each other, but the distance prevented them from touching. Tentatively they asked after each other's injuries. As soon as Marilyn was allowed out of bed she went to David and sat on a chair next to him. Their hands met for the first time in ages. No words were necessary.

Soon Marilyn was well enough to leave, but the doctors insisted that David needed to spend at least a further two weeks in hospital. She phoned her mother and the children to tell them about the accident, and reassured them that she and David would soon be home. Then she rented a room close to the hospital, so that she could be with David while he recovered.

With few distractions other than the medical staff, they began to talk. At first they talked about the shock of the accident, how fortunate they were to have survived, and shared their memories before finally waking. They discussed their children. They were concerned that the tense atmosphere between them, followed by their trip away, would cause their children distress.

Then talk turned to their marriage.

'I'm sorry I hurt you,' David said softly, as he looked down.

'I was at fault too,' she said, taking his hand. 'I didn't devote enough time to you. I was stressed, trying to manage work, the children and the house...and I didn't give you the love you needed.'

He nodded. 'That's true but I acted stupidly. I should've told you how I was feeling instead of falling into Gina's arms. I won't be seeing her again...I promise.'

They kissed and Marilyn wiped away a few tears. She took David's hand. 'I'll see to it that you don't,' she said with a smile. 'Now that the business is doing well, I'm going to be home more and spend time with the children.'

When David was discharged, they hired a car. They drove home slowly, enjoying being together, stopping for a day or two at small towns they hadn't visited before.

In spite of their pain and suffering, and damage to the car, David and Marilyn gave and received far more from their trip than a holiday at the beach could have offered them.

Golden Riches

After work, Geoff stopped at the local pub for a fortifying drink before going home.

He and Cheryl had been high school sweethearts with romantic dreams of their future together. They were married at twenty and their three children followed soon after, but marriage hadn't followed their dream. Financial strain, the pressure of work and parenting took its toll. With them both working and the children to care for, their old friendships fell away. They bickered endlessly and had lost their joy in being together. In moments of anger and resentment, Geoff had threatened to leave, and Cheryl did not attempt to dissuade him.

While Geoff was drinking his beer, relaxing for the first time that day, he overheard two men near him discussing their riches gained from gold prospecting and the nuggets they had found at a reopened old gold mine.

He hurried home to tell Cheryl what he'd heard. As he told her his news she began to walk away, and replied cynically, 'It's all very well, but there's no quick fix for our money problems.'

Geoff wiped his brow as his frustration rose. 'At least hear me out. This might be the chance we've been hoping for.'

'We've tried all your harebrained schemes in the past, and they didn't work out. I'm trying to be reasonable, but we don't know a thing about gold mining. These guys might've been talking a load of rubbish.'

'Okay I get it, Cheryl. I'll do some research, ask around, but you have to admit it's a great idea.'

She raised her eyebrows in disbelief. He nodded and walked towards the fridge to grab a beer.

Nothing could put Geoff off his new interest in prospecting. He read all he could find about it on the Internet and joined a library, to read the recommended books. Then he joined a prospecting club that met fortnightly. Cheryl noticed the effort Geoff was devoting to learning about prospecting and relented. Perhaps there is something in it after all, she thought. They had long discussions over dinner about his discoveries, and she began to encourage him. Now that they had a common interest other than their children, they talked to each other more often, and their arguing ceased.

When Geoff was almost ready to attempt prospecting, experienced members of the club suggested he visit a disused gold mine a short distance away. The following week, he took two days off work and drove to a town close to the mine. At the local library and historical society he viewed plans of the mine, and read newspaper archives covering the history of gold discovery in the area. He made a point of eating with the locals and tapping into some of their knowledge. The visit confirmed the positive information he had been given about the mine. He drove home a happy man keen to apply for a mining permit.

Cheryl and Geoff drank a toast to their future. They were both working, and they only had weekends for prospecting, but fortunately, Cheryl's mother liked the idea of having the children to stay and agreed to care for them for at least some of the time they would be away.

Organisation for their first weekend away began in earnest. They dipped into their "rainy day" savings to buy a metal detector, picks, shovels and other equipment. Cheryl borrowed a tent and sleeping bags from friends.

They left for the old mine late one Friday afternoon. The sky was striped with tangerine when they found their site on the hill amongst scattered tents, caravans and makeshift sheds. Before dark their tent was erected, their equipment in place.

That weekend, they used their metal detector for the first time. A neighbour watching their amateurish efforts gave them some tips on how best to use it. Soon they were holding the detector close to the ground and swinging it slowly to cover an area. After several hours of short signals, the detector beeped furiously indicating something under the surface. Eagerly they raked the leaves and grass, and began to dig. Unfortunately, all they found was a large piece of charcoal.

During week days, they talked about nothing else but finding gold, and all the joy it would bring them. Each weekend at the mine they became more practiced at digging, prying rocks loose, and carting away rubble. It was hard work and they were exhausted by the end of the day. They continued panning and sifting carefully, but found nothing of value. Friendly prospectors on the hill visited, and shared stories of their hard work, and their finds. On Saturday nights, everyone working the old mine met at the local hotel for dinner and drinks. Geoff and Cheryl were invited to join them and had fun for the first time in years.

One sunny weekend after backbreaking work, Geoff came across a solid slab of rock with a shimmering seam. He called out to Cheryl excitedly, 'Quickly, come and have a look at this!'

She saw the shining speckles and grinned. 'At last! It could be the real thing.'

'It looks good to me!' he said, giving her a hug.

They began the gruelling job of digging the seam from the rock. That night, they continued working using a spotlight. By morning, they had freed a piece of shining rock and sifted away the rubble. After washing the rock in the nearby stream, they held it up to the light and admired its yellow lustre.

Cheryl stroked the rock. 'Beautiful, isn't it.'

Geoff eyes glowed with delight. 'It's what we've been waiting for.'

They hurried into the town to have their find assayed. When the assayer walked towards them with a downcast expression, they knew something was wrong. They moved closer to each other as they listened to his words.

'What you have here is a large chunk of iron pyrite…what we call "fool's gold". Unfortunately it's worthless. It sparkles like gold and dupes thousands of prospectors each year.'

Cheryl couldn't hide her tears of disappointment. They had spent so much money, worked so hard, and discovered nothing of value.

'I should've known it would turn out like this,' Geoff said, walking towards the car.

Cheryl kept walking for a while without replying.

Geoff kicked a stone on the sidewalk. 'I had huge hopes pinned on a find. I can't help being disappointed.'

Cheryl put her arm around his shoulder. 'I've had enough, but I'm prepared to keep going…and give it another try if you're set on it.'

He shook his head. 'Nah! It seemed like such a great opportunity,' he said, looking towards the hillside with a sigh.

'We knew that we were taking a chance and it's been fun doing it together,' she said.

'Yeah, I guess it has been fun. We've tried our best and I reckon it's time to move on.'

They sold all their equipment at a loss, packed their things and set off for home. In the car, they were both quiet at first, mulling over their losses. But within a short while they were chatting, regaling stories about their experiences, and the people they had met while prospecting.

When they arrived home, Cheryl took Geoff's hand. 'Don't worry, we'll manage. I'll do some extra hours. We'll recover most of our money.'

'Sticking to a budget will help too. I spend far too impulsively,' he said.

Cheryl nodded. 'We need to be more careful with our money, but on the plus side we've found something valuable.'

'You're right. Prospecting taught us to talk to each other again and work together. No gold could equal that find...and we've made some good friends too.'

Cheryl nodded and smiled. 'Let's pick up the children and then visit my mum. We'll have a lot to tell them.'

Laura's Birthday

It was Friday morning and Laura's birthday. She waited for Karel's loving kiss, a gift from him, or a card. But, that year there was nothing. He left for work with a breezy goodbye as he did every day. He had forgotten her birthday, or so it seemed. She waited. Perhaps he would send her flowers at work, or surprise her with a booking for dinner at a fancy restaurant. By the end of the day, her birthday was almost over with no words of love or celebration. She made excuses for him. He had a new job that kept him busier than usual, and he brought work home over the weekend. But, she couldn't help wondering if something had changed - if he still loved her. He hadn't forgotten her birthday before.

By the evening, her excuses for his forgetfulness evaporated. For his birthday, she had made him a chocolate cake, and bought him an expensive gift. Though she was hurt by his forgetfulness she decided not to remind him.

That Saturday, Karel went to a football match with his friends. After a week at work, Laura's household chores had banked up. Though she liked a tidy house, she decided to put the tasks aside until later.

The day was warm, perfect for a walk in the nature reserve near her home. She walked at an even pace, enjoying the sunlight until she reached the creek that ran through the park. She turned away to avoid looking at the water, walking past it as briskly as she could. As a child she had almost drowned in a river, and ever since then, the sea, lakes and rivers brought back the unpleasant memory.

After an hour of walking with a breeze spurring her on, she stopped to rest. She sighed with pleasure at the glorious view of trees and undulating hills. As she relaxed, her eyes closed and she began to daydream.

She was in a forest when she came across stone steps. Though she had no idea where the steps led, she was curious, and went down them. At the bottom of the steps, a closed wooden door stood before her. Intuitively, she knew that she was meant to open it. When she turned the door's brass knob it opened onto a rambling garden. She noticed how tiny she had become. Huge, dazzling flowers surrounded her, large leaves swayed in the wind and wild tendrils grasped enormous trees. Even the grass was as high as her waist.

A white dove surrounded by an aura of light sat on the branch of the tree above her. After watching her for a while, the dove fluttered down and settled on her shoulder. It pecked her ear for attention. Then it flew around her in widening circles, beckoning her to follow it through the garden. As doves had visited her before in her dreams to bring her messages, she followed it until she reached a rock pool sparkling in the light. The dove hovered as if asking her to stay.

One look at the water, and Laura took a step back in fear. It took all her courage to prevent her from running off. She watched the dove dive into the shimmering pool with its bobbing water lilies and swaying rushes. It ruffled its feathers with joy and playfully sprinkled her with water. Delighting in the cool, she smiled. 'After the dove dried itself in the sunlight, it flew around her once more, waiting for her to follow. By now, she had resumed her adult size as the dove took her past perfumed shrubs and flowering trees.

On a tall branch, she noticed a second white dove. The birds greeted each other in low coos. They cuddled and their beaks touched, as they pecked each other lightly on the neck. She watched the loving couple amazed.

Sounds of walkers talking and laughing woke Laura. She yawned, stretched, and then walked home at a leisurely pace. This time when she passed the creek, she glanced at it, but didn't linger. Somehow, she was slightly less afraid of the water.

Karel was lounging on the sofa watching television when she returned. As they sat together chatting, she thought of her daydream and the loving birds. How much she loved him, she thought. She ought to have told him that he had upset her.

'There's been something upsetting me that I need to tell you,' she said hesitantly.

Karel turned, and looked up at her with a worried expression. 'What is it? Tell me.'

'You forgot my birthday this week...and...'

'I thought your birthday was this coming Monday.' He looked shocked. 'I'm so sorry darling. I don't know how I mixed up the days. You know that I love you far too much to upset you.' He put his arm around her and kissed her.

'Don't worry about it...but I thought that I should tell you.'

'I'm glad you did.' He was quiet for a moment. 'I was thinking of going out for dinner to celebrate next week, so why don't we do that tonight instead?'

'That's a great idea!'

They enjoyed a delicious meal, touched hands and kissed. When the coffee arrived, Karel put his hand into his pocket and took out a small box. 'This is the birthday gift I bought to give you on Monday. 'Happy birthday my darling!'

The box contained a magnificent pearl necklace. 'Oh Karel, it's beautiful. I love it,' she said kissing him. 'Thank you.' She placed it around her neck. 'How does it look?' she asked, smiling.

'You look beautiful.'

Once they were home, Karel put his arm around her. 'Another glass of wine before bed? It's Sunday tomorrow and we can sleep a bit later,' he said.

They were sipping their second glass, when Laura heard a few taps at the window. She pushed back the net curtain and saw a white dove. She went outside to see the dove more clearly, but it had flown away. On the doormat was a silky, white feather. She smiled as she bent to pick it up. As she stroked the feather, she thought of the two loving doves in her daydream. 'You've sent me a message,' she whispered.

The Stars

It was Sunday. The house was still, the atmosphere tense. Kaitlyn was seated on the sofa, two-thirds of the way through a block of chocolate, while pretending to read her book. The only sounds were the drip of the laundry tap and the trill of cicadas in the tall trees. Corey sat opposite, sipping a beer while flicking through messages on his iPad. A large black dog lay at his feet. It was unusual for the couple to be alone in their large house, but this weekend Liam, their youngest child, was away at a school camp and Ava was sleeping over with friends.

Once they had eaten their early snack of sandwiches with coffee, they hardly talked. Kaitlyn recognized Corey's familiar signs of withdrawal, and knew that no amount of chatter would entice him to talk to her. Lately she was feeling lonely. Corey was there in the room with her, but his mind was somewhere else. She ate the last of her chocolate and put her book down. With some force she threw the ball of scrunched leftover foil into a corner. Enough of this, she thought. As she stood, she glanced through the open glass doors. It was a clear, warm night with the stir of a breeze.

'Let's take Romulus for a walk,' she suggested.

'Good idea. Let's get out of the house.' Corey gulped down the last of his beer.

The dog's ear tweaked at the word "walk" and he stood, with tail wagging, a whine of expectation escaping his large frame.

As soon as they were past their front gate, Romulus pulled on the lead.

'Hang on there, boy.' Corey gave the dog a quick pat. 'You can run as soon as we get to the park.'

The couple walked on in silence. When they neared the park, Corey untied the lead. They heard the dog's joyful bark as they watched his dark shape disappear.

'He certainly needs his exercise,' she said with a laugh.

'As much as he can get,' he replied, as they walked up a slope.

They stopped at a viewing spot they had visited often when they were younger. Kaitlyn took a deep breath, and inhaled the scent of the night. She looked up at the sky peppered with stars and the crescent moon. 'Incredible isn't it? Look up there, the Milky Way,' she pointed. 'And the pinpoints of light from the houses below.'

'I can just make out Canopus over in the South-East,' he said excitedly. 'And Orion's saucepan with its three stars.'

'It's a pity we didn't bring the binoculars tonight.'

'So glad you suggested a walk,' he said, as he put his arm around her shoulder.

She nodded. 'Me too. We should do this more often.'

'I've been grumpy lately…sorry…but I've had a lot on my mind. I'm trying to get a new idea going at work and it hasn't been easy. People prefer the old ways and don't take easily to new ways of doing things.'

'We all get stuck at times,' Kaitlyn said with a laugh. 'But you should've shared it with me.'

'I know…I tend to get frustrated and clam up when I shouldn't.'

'True. I wish you'd talk more. I can see you're stressed, but I don't know how to help.'

'I need to talk about my ideas at work too…explain more of my thinking to everyone,' Corey murmured.

'At home and at work,' she said with a smile.

They sat on a tree trunk enjoying the view.

She sighed. 'Isn't this magical?'

He drew her closer and kissed her. 'Love you!'

'Love you too,' she said, as she gently stroked Corey's hair.

'Let's call Romulus and head for home,' he said softly.

'Good idea. The children are away and we have the house to ourselves,' she replied, taking Corey's hand.

Young Love

I noticed Vic at an anatomy lecture during my first term at university. His hazel eyes and full mouth attracted me. He caught my gaze and smiled at me. After the lecture we chatted about our hopes of qualifying as physiotherapists. The next day we had coffee together, and then we met after lectures the following week. We laughed a lot and had so much to talk about that we started to see each other regularly. I fell for Vic in a big way and was relaxed in his company. I was surprised because I hadn't felt like that about any of the guys I had dated before. Being together was fun, whether we went to a movie, for a walk, bought fish and chips, or were just messing about. Our tastes and ideas were similar. We had detailed and analytical discussions about everything we attended, from exhibitions, to philosophical and political lectures, and experimental plays. It was silly, but we even made up our own language, and had a phase of dressing in the same colours.

Our course was tough and we helped each with our studies. We were both living at home. Vic's parents and mine seemed happy enough about our relationship. Within a short while we became part of each other's families. I had a younger sister and brother who adored Vic and treated him as an older brother. Vic's two brothers had left home already. His older sister Angie was fun and an excellent cook.

When I made my decision to go to university, I had hoped it would be an adventure, a time of experimentation, increased independence and growing up. I had expected to date lots of guys without being serious about any of them, but, I hadn't banked on meeting Vic.

Our first year together was like a fairy tale. On our first anniversary we celebrated our love for each other at the lake. Early in our relationship, the lake with its magnificent view of the water lapping the foothills of the mountain became our special spot. Later we had dinner at a restaurant in a hotel in the city. As I hadn't bought Vic a gift, I was taken aback when he presented me with a silver friendship ring. The day was so romantic that I dreamed about it for weeks.

I guess things would've been perfect, if Vic hadn't wanted to be with me all the time, to share everything with me. I felt consumed by our relationship. I had lost touch with my girlfriends, missed our late parties, and long gossipy talks. Though I loved him and wanted to be with him, I was losing my separateness and independence.

I was determined to do something about it. I attended yoga classes and spent time with my friends once more. Painting had been a hobby for years. I joined an art group at the university. My large, brightly coloured and expressive paintings were a surprise. Vic found them a bit overpowering, but my teacher was encouraging. Initially, Vic wasn't happy about my show of independence, but after a few discussions, he accepted it. He even went out with his mates as he had before meeting me. With more balance in our relationship, we remained together happily through our first three years of study.

In our fourth and final year, I noticed changes in Vic. He no longer had his heart in his studies. When he talked about the future, it wasn't about his career, but about travel, mountain climbing or learning to fly. He was studying less and missed some of the practical sessions with patients at the hospital. The sessions were essential to our course. In working with patients we put all the theory we had learned into practice. I tried to encourage him, but he had a variety of excuses.

By then, I had become an involved and committed student. Study was no longer a chore and I wanted to learn as much as possible. I found new ideas and ways of helping people both stimulating and exciting. I looked forward to the days I spent working in the hospital wards and was learning all the time. It became clear to me that once I was qualified I would work in a hospital.

Everyone we knew thought of us as a couple and it began to bother me. Neither of us were ready for a long term relationship. The fun part of being together simply evaporated when our final exams neared. We argued for the first time, both pulling in different directions.

We both passed our finals, and after the stress of exams was over we continued spending time together. We were at the lake enjoying the crisp autumn air and the vibrantly coloured landscape, when he surprised me by saying that he wasn't sure if he was suited to physiotherapy, and that he wanted to work in another field for a few years. The biggest bombshell hit me two days later, when he told me that his family were moving from Canberra to Sydney. As he hadn't found work, he decided to go with them. He insisted that distance between us was only a three to four hour drive, but it seemed far to me.

Once he left, we talked daily, sent each other texts, videos and surprise gifts. Most weekends and holidays we spent together, but somehow it didn't work. As soon as he could afford the rent for an apartment in Sydney, we parted. As difficult as it was, we agreed that the break would probably be positive for both of us. Either we would find other partners, or we would find our way back together with stronger commitment.

Life without Vic was a struggle at first. I thought of him in all my free moments, wondered what he was doing, kept returning to his Facebook page, and longed to phone him, just to hear his voice again. Then I found my feet, determined to experience all the challenges, new experiences and growing up that I had intended before meeting him. I read *War and Peace*, everything by Jane Austin, Hemingway and Steinbeck, and dipped into the philosophy of Sartre, Marx and Kierkegaard. I spent time with friends, and met new people. When study allowed, I went to the theatre, films, and lectures on topics that had not interested me before. I cut my hair, stopped dyeing it blonde, and wore simple comfortable clothing. I no longer cared what others thought or said about me. My sense of independence blossomed. There were other guys in my life too. After dating several, I was drawn to Max, a dashingly handsome artist. We saw each other constantly for about a year until I heard he had been dating another woman. My hurt turned me off guys for months, but I was growing up, and learning to be more selective about the men I dated.

Almost three years after breaking up, Vic and I found our way back to each other. He was attending a study course in Canberra, and gave me a call. We met for a drink at one of our old haunts. After a few awkward moments, we connected as if we hadn't been apart. There was no need for lengthy decisions. We wanted to be together, and whatever the obstacles, we knew that this time we would make it work. Vic had travelled, dated other women and worked casually. I was surprised that he had returned to his profession and was enjoying working in a physiotherapy practice.

We were friends as well as lovers, and discussed everything, sharing our thoughts about events of the day, what food to eat, and where we would stay. We rented an old house and bought a dog we called Candy. The need for adventure and stimulation had not decreased for either of us, but this time we wanted to satisfy it together.

After much discussion, we bought a minivan. At the end of the year we both took leave, and with Candy, set out in the van to explore. We drove hundreds of kilometers, camping along the way. We walked, swam, climbed, tried sky diving, and went to museums in towns we had not visited before. When we returned to work, we settled back into a routine, knowing that being together was what really counted. We are still together and our love for each other hasn't diminished.

Love Letters

Kathy and Damien were living together. Their small, apartment suited Damien when he lived alone, but with two of them living there it was cramped and messy, with piles of books, boxes and clothing scattered on the floor. Kathy was a teacher and Damien was a pilot with the Australian Defense Force, often away flying missions in the Middle East. While he was away Kathy was constantly in his thoughts.

Kathy loved Damien and was lonely when he wasn't with her. She was proud of him, but longed to spend more time with him. Flying over areas at war was dangerous. Though he was an excellent pilot, she worried about his safety. Reports of friendly fire, air crashes and technical glitches concerned her.

She wanted her home tidy and large enough to entertain a few friends, or to put up her easel to paint on evenings after work, while Damien was away. She searched until she found a suitable spacious and airy apartment. Damien liked the apartment and agreed to the move as long as she handled all the financial arrangements, and did most of the packing.

While Damien was away, Kathy packed their possessions, allowing herself to dream, and almost believe, that their move to a comfortable apartment might encourage him to be at home more.

She was sorting books in a bulging, antique bookcase that had belonged to her grandmother, when an old, leather photo album slid from the shelf and fell to the floor. She placed the faded, album on the bed and turned the pages. Photographs of her aunts and uncles in their youth stared at her. She noticed a photograph of her great grandmother, Jessie, who had died before she was born. Jessie was about twenty in the photograph, slim with long hair tied back and wispy curls framing her pretty face.

As Kathy paged through the album, she found two buff envelopes addressed to her great grandmother. She was intrigued and about to open one of letters, when the phone rang. It was a friend, suggesting that they eat out that night. While Damien was away, escape from eating alone was always appealing. Before heading for the bedroom to change her clothes, she absentmindedly left the letters on the hall table to read later.

Damien retuned in time for the move to the new apartment. He was about to lift the hall table and carry it to the moving van when he noticed the two letters. He picked up one of them, assuming it couldn't be personal if it was lying on the table. He noticed the date, 15th September1914. Carefully he spread the brittle, yellowed paper covered in copperplate on the table, and read it.

Dearest Jessica,

It pains me to write this letter to you, my love, as I think of you constantly. I am sad to tell you that I have to leave you. With black war clouds looming and our country threatened, my duty is to serve my country.

Who would have believed that we are now at war, and that within just a few weeks the seas will no longer be safe to travel? By the time you receive this letter, my dearest, I will have begun my training. Within a short while, I expect to receive a call that my regiment will be joining others leaving for the front. I will defend my country proudly and with every ounce of my being.

Although I care so much for you, I believe that it will be for the best that I fade from your life. War is cruel and unpredictable and I do not think it fair to ask you to wait for me. You talked often of Barry Kegan, and that he had asked you to marry him. He is medically unfit to fight for his country, but from what you have told me of him, he seems to be a fair man who makes a good living. Most importantly, he appears to love and care for you.

Whatever God has in store for us both, I know we will remain in each other's hearts. I will write to you again if I return from the war. I shouldn't ask this of you, but as you go about your daily life, think of me from time to time.

May God bless you!

Your ever-loving,

Jonathan.

The letter was from another era, but the depth of feeling touched Damien. He knew the anxious feeling in his guts every time he left for service overseas only too well. He wasn't in open combat now, and there was less danger than there had been during his service in Afghanistan, but the fear of not returning was real. He had found his own ways of shutting it out. Alcohol helped in the short-term, but he couldn't drink if he was due to fly, as it dulled his concentration. He was fatalistic about death, but capture by the enemy was something he would not allow himself to even consider. That morning, he had received an email about his next period of overseas service in two weeks. He had not told Kathy about it yet, as he knew she would be upset about another parting.

Curiosity drove him to open the second letter dated 6th December 1918.

Dearest Jessica,

I am writing to you from the train to London. How I survived the war I do not know, but I am one of the lucky ones. It goes without saying, that when guns were firing around me and bullets flying, my thoughts of you gave me courage. It is best that I write nothing of the awful things I have seen, and the dreadful deeds I have committed in the name of war.

I learned much about myself in those dark moments. My military training was put to good use, and with God on our side we won at least some of our battles.

As soon as I returned, I discovered that you had indeed accepted Barry Kegan's proposal, and that you now have a child. My hope is that you are well and happy.

I have loved you all this time, and I will think of you and hold you dear to my heart no matter where my life takes me. A secret part of me had hoped that you had waited for me to return from the war, but when your marriage was confirmed I became engaged to a childhood sweetheart, Simone Harrison. She is a fine looking woman from a good family. We care for each other, but our relationship lacks the love that you and I once shared. I dare not allow my mind to stray to our moments together.

Unfortunately, you and I met at the wrong time, but you will always be in my heart.

May God bless you.

Your ever-loving,

Jonathan

Damien wiped his moist eyes with his sleeve. He sighed, suddenly overcome with tiredness. He thought about his role in the Middle East. Somehow, he no longer looked forward to the sorties with a rush of adrenaline. He had always enjoyed flying, but he admitted to himself that his missions were extremely dangerous. What distressed him most was that so many civilians had been unavoidably killed from the sky. He thought about war, the destruction of nations, cities, families and relationships, and that he was part of it. It was no longer what he wanted to do. This overseas mission would be his last. Though he would miss his mates, it was time for him to leave and spend more time with Kathy. He loved her and wanted to marry her, and felt sure it was what Kathy wanted too. The move to a new place would be positive. He felt certain of that.

An Ending that Led to a New Beginning

I have been divorced from Jordan for three years. When we first split up, I felt as if I had fallen into the blackest hole, but now my life has turned around. I'm living with someone who respects and genuinely loves me. My story is not unusual. So many men and women find themselves in the same situation, but it's what one does about it that counts.

After twenty-two years of marriage to Jordan, I discovered that he was cheating on me. It was something he said that didn't add up that gave me the clue. When I looked through his wallet and found credit card slips to hotels and restaurants we had not been to together, that had nothing to do with his work, my suspicions were confirmed. When I confronted him with my findings, he cried as he admitted that he had been with another woman. I had not seen him in tears since the birth of Mia, our first born. He told me the other woman "didn't mean a thing to him…it was just for sex," and that "I was the one and only he really loved." He promised to stop seeing her, but I didn't trust him. The thought of him being with her played over and over in my head.

I decided to make some changes. I no longer tried to please him by making his favorite meals or wearing the clothes he liked. I wasn't trying to be mean, but my loving and caring feelings for him had dried up. When my spontaneous hugs and kisses stopped, he withdrew and we hardly talked. It was scary having to admit to myself that our marriage was dead. After all, I was in my forties with two children. Like many other women who thought of leaving their husbands, the emotional and physical health of my children, as well as having sufficient money to care for them and myself, were my biggest concern. For a while I pretended I was managing, but I was miserable. If I had been a vindictive person I could've paid him back with an affair, but I wasn't like that. Being with another man was the last thing I wanted right then.

I did not tell a soul about our troubles. It was an old friend Janice, who noticed that I was not what she called "my usual bubbly self". Between sobs, I told her the truth about our marriage. She listened without interrupting.

'A job…going back to work will solve some of your problems. Then you'll have the money and confidence to leave him,' she said, and gave me a hug.

I thought about Janice's advice for days. I had been a secretary to a solicitor before having my children, but lately bosses had personal assistants who were highly computer literate. My computer skills were fine for home use, but not at the level required in a busy office. The idea of having to upgrade my skills didn't appeal to me, and jobs were not that easy to find either.

I let it slip for longer, hoping things between us would change. It was Mia, my sixteen year old daughter who shook me with her insight.

'Mum, I can tell that you're not happy, that you're not the person you were when Ralf and I were young,' she said. 'You and dad hardly talk to each other lately, and when you two do talk, it's to argue.'

I was astounded, and tried not to cry.

'If you're staying together for us…don't. You've got your own life to lead, and we can handle a split if it has to be that way.'

After our talk I didn't sleep for a few nights. She was right of course.

Mia encouraged me to look for a suitable computer course. Finding a course was easy enough, but forcing myself to start it was harder. Eventually I attended classes every week and practiced at home until I was ready to apply for a job. Jordan said that it was a good idea that I was keeping myself busy, but he didn't realise that I was actually planning to return to the workforce, so that I could be in a position to leave him.

It was a struggle to find a job at my age without recent experience. After countless attempts, I landed a job with a solicitor at a salary higher than I had expected. In the past, young assistants had let him down and he wanted an older and more responsible person. I was thrilled.

During that year at work, I was tired at night, bought a lot of take away food, and went to bed early. Jordon and I spent very little time together during the week, and on the weekend he played golf. My boss was pleased with my work, and told me so. Every Friday I went out with some of my new work mates. My life had improved.

It was time for me to move on. Over a weekend, I told Jordan that I wanted to leave him. He hadn't seen it coming, though he should've. He begged me not to leave, but I'd had enough. After he moved out, we saw a solicitor. There were no arguments, and I was left with an amount I thought was fair.

When it was final, I panicked. What if I felt alone and miserable without him? The younger children would move away soon. Mia was talking of sharing a house with her boyfriend.

Well, within a few weeks of our divorce, my phone started ringing. The news of my marriage break up was out. I was asked out on dates like a teenager. This was not something I had anticipated. After many evenings with men who didn't interest or attract me, I met Stephen. He is a little older than me, but I like his looks, and well, I'm biased. I'm happy and in love again. Perhaps even more importantly, we are good friends, and I respect and trust him. There's no point in saying I should've left Jordon earlier, but I wasn't ready then.

For Young Children
(3-6 Years)

Late at Night

Chloe and Aria were three and a half, and identical twins who liked to do everything together. They looked the same and only their family and friends could tell them apart. They had the same moods, the same scared feelings, and sometimes the same dreams.

They were happy during the day, but at night they were scared of the dark. At night, the Giants and Little Nasties visited. Even the night light that their mother bought for them didn't help. Their beds were side by side and as soon as Mum and Dad went to bed, Chloe crawled into Aria's bed. They lay together cuddling… waited and listened.

"Crackle, crackle" were the sounds in the walls and ceiling when the weather changed. "Bang, Bang' was the noise in the water pipes. The noises were a warning that the Giants were visiting. While the twins slept the heavy Giants sat on the twins with a "plomp" and gave them sore tummies.

The Little Nasties visited when the wind blew the tree outside, so that its branches scratched the window, and the water pipes went "thump, thump". The twins shivered as they waited for the Little Nasties with their sharp pointed feet to walk over them. "Prink, prink" they went, as they threw the warm covers off the twins' beds.

Eventually Chloe and Aria fell asleep. When the morning light shone through the curtain, Chloe woke and went back to her own bed. Their parents had no idea that the girls were sleeping together most of the night, or how scared they were.

One night, when the air was hot and the moon shone into their room, the twins were almost asleep when a strange thing happened. Their window was open with the breeze blowing the curtain back making "swish, swish" noises. The twins listened out for visitors, but all they could hear was the sound of a dog barking and frogs croaking.

Then a golden creature flew into the room.

'Look, look…there's a fairy in the room,' whispered Chloe. 'Can you see its pretty wings?'

Aria looked up at the fairy. 'I wonder why it's here.'

The fairy talked in a sweet, soft voice. 'I've come to help you both,' it said, as it swirled around the room.'

Chloe clapped her hands. Aria waited and watched.

'I'm here to get rid of the Giants and the Little Nasties that visit you at night. I promise to be back with my plans soon, but please be patient…it may take me a while.'

The next morning, Chloe smiled happily. 'If we get rid of our horrid visitors we won't be so scared at night, or so tired in the morning.'

'It was just a silly dream, Chloe,' Aria said. 'The Giants and the Little Nasties will always be here.'

'Don't be so silly Aria!' Chloe replied crossly. 'We both saw the fairy and I'm sure she'll help us, but she asked us to be patient.'

The twins waited and waited for the fairy to return. When almost a month had passed and the moon was full and round again, a golden light shone. The curtains went "swish, swish" and the fairy flitted into the room.

Chloe pinched her twin. 'See, I told you the fairy would come back.'

'I'm going to make sure that the Giants and the Nasties will never ever bother you again,' the fairy said, as she fluttered her wings.

Chloe smiled. 'Thank you, thank you!'

Aria muttered her thanks too.

'This is a secret, so don't tell anyone,' the fairy put her finger to lips and whispered. 'Special helpers will get rid of your night visitors, but they won't know why.'

The twins looked at each other wondering what would happen.

'Can you guess who the special helpers will be?' the fairy asked.

'The nice lady next door,' Aria said.

'The old man who lives across the road,' Chloe suggested.

After lots of tries, neither of the twins could guess correctly.

'Well then, it's going to be a lovely surprise,' the fairy said, and flew off into the moonlight.

Later that week, the twins' mother sat at the breakfast table rubbing her head. 'I had a strange dream last night. I saw a fairy in the moonlight. I haven't seen fairies since I was your age,' she said to the twins with a smile. 'I saw them often at night and loved them. It was strange having a fairy visit me again after all this time. She danced and sang to me, but I can't remember any of it this morning.' Their mother ate her breakfast and yawned loudly. 'I'm so tired this morning. After my dream the noises in the walls, and the water pipes thumping kept me from going back to sleep.'

'The noises in this old house are dreadful. I'm going to phone someone today to get rid of them,' their father said.

The twins looked at each other and giggled, but didn't say a word.

A few days, later a big van drove up to the house and a tall man in overalls carrying a toolbox rang the doorbell. He had come to fix the noises. For a whole week he repaired the walls, ceilings and water pipes.

After the repair man left, the twins listened for their night visitors, but all was quiet. Cloe and Aria slept in their own beds. They were not afraid of the night again.

Chloe opened the window in their room and the two girls looked up towards the moon. 'Thank you, little fairy,' they said together.

Crystal, Alba and Blackie

Two fluffy white cats, Crystal and Alba lived in a big house with a Mom, Dad and two young children, Alan and Robert. The children loved their cats. They fed the cats, groomed them every day, played with them and petted them. As well as their usual food, the children gave the cats treats and snacks. Each night, Crystal slept on Alan's bed, and Alba slept on Robert's.

'We're such lucky cats. Our owners love us and feed us delicious food,' Crystal said to Alba.

'Yes, we are very lucky,' Alba said licking her paws after her meal. 'We are happy here and couldn't ask for more.'

When Alan, the eldest child turned five, there was a party for his birthday, with cake and presents. Dad came home that night with a large box, a gift for Alan. When Alan opened the box a small black dog jumped out.

Alan was thrilled and hugged his dad. 'He's beautiful! Thank you! I couldn't have a nicer present for my birthday…and I'll share him with Robert, and with you and mum too.'

'I know that you love Crystal and Alba, but you wanted a dog too. I saw this puppy and thought you'd like him. It will be your job to look after him and train him,' Dad said.

'The cats won't like the dog at first, so be careful to keep them apart for a while,' Mum said.

'What are you going to call him?' Dad asked.

'Blackie,' Alan said, cuddling the puppy.

'Yes, Blackie suits him,' Dad said with a smile.

Crystal and Alba didn't like the smell of Blackie at all. He jumped around a lot, made loud noises and wagged his tail. They didn't understand the puppy, as cats only wag their tails when they are cross or upset. Blackie wasn't as clean as they were, and made big, smelly messes on the floor. The boys spent a lot of time cleaning up after him and trying to house train him.

'Disgusting!' Crystal said. 'He needs a litter box.'

After a while, Blackie learned to go outside and didn't mess the floor any longer. Alan and Robert played with him and petted him in the same way they had once petted their cats. They fed Blackie and gave him snacks. But sometimes they forgot to feed Crystal and Alba until they cried for food. The cats were upset and no longer slept on the boys' beds.

'The children don't love and appreciate us now,' Alba said sadly. 'And the food isn't as good as it was before.'

'We should teach them a lesson,' Crystal said.

Alba licked her paws and nodded in agreement.

The next day, the two cats hid at the back of the linen closet. When the boys came home from school, they called the cats, but they didn't come.

'Where could they be?' Alan said, after searching through the house and garden.

Robert looked worried. 'Do you think they've have run away?'

Even Blackie began to search for them.

When Mum came home she hunted for the cats too. 'I've found them,' she shouted. 'Give them some special food and tell them how much you love them. The two of you gave Blackie a lot of attention and forgot about your old friends. They are letting you know how upset they are.'

The boys were so pleased to see Alba and Crystal that they fed them chicken. Then they hugged and stroked them. The cats purred loudly. Blackie wagged his tail, and the cats understood at last that he was pleased to see them too.

Poppy's Cushion

Poppy the Labrador was chocolate brown and had beautiful, big dark eyes. She was Tara and Gabe's dog and they loved her. They fed her, threw the ball for her, and played hide and seek with her. After dinner when they watched television, Poppy cuddled up between them on the couch, and enjoyed being petted.

It was Tara who first noticed that Poppy had a fat tummy. In a week or two her tummy grew even fatter. Mum said that soon there would be puppies. Tara and Gabe were excited and wondered what the puppies would look like, and how many there would be.

Dad said that Poppy needed a special place where she could have her puppies and look after them. The children hunted in the garage for the right box. The first one they found was too small, the next far too big. At last, they found a box that was the perfect size. Gabe cut a hole in the side of it for Poppy to move in and out easily. But, Poppy didn't like the box. She sniffed it and walked away.

'Maybe it isn't comfortable enough for her,' Tara said. 'I'll put an old towel inside the box. Maybe she will like it then.'

Poppy sat on the towel once, and walked off. She didn't wag her tail as she did when she was happy.

'I think we should give her our big cushion. Then she'll be comfortable,' Tara said.

'I love sitting on that cushion, but I love Poppy more,' Gabe said.

So the children put their cushion in the box. This time Poppy went into the box and fell asleep inside. A few days later, six tiny puppies were born.

Gabe and Tara watched Poppy feed and care for the puppies. They were pleased that they had made the dog they loved comfortable and happy by giving her something special of their own.

The Pond

Once upon a time, a green frog lived on a big pond in a lovely garden with lots of flowers and trees. At night when he came out, he ate grubs and insects that lived around the water. Then he played by jumping about. When he was tired, he lay on a water lily leaf and relaxed as he drifted across the pond.

"Crack, crack", he croaked, enjoying himself.

The frog liked the rain, but that year, the rain didn't visit his garden often. The flowers and grasses died, and the hot sun burned up the water in the pond. Insects that lived around the water flew away, and the frog was hungry.

"Craaaack, craaaak," the green frog croaked sadly.

When the pond dried up to a small puddle and no more rain came, the frog cried and cried.

'I have to do something,' he said to himself.

So, he hopped under the trees to search for water, but there was none. He hopped further from his home into the bushes, but he could not find water there either. Then he hopped to parts of the garden he had not visited before. He was scared. Maybe the cats that prowled at night would chase him, and even try to eat him. He told himself to keep searching for water, but to hop slowly and carefully like his Mama had taught him.

He hopped and hopped until he was close to the house where people lived. At first he saw only brick walls. Then he heard a tiny trickle of water saying "drip, drip". The sound was coming from a tap on the side of the house. In no time he found it, and sat under the cool water. He was hungry, and that night he found a few insects buzzing near the water. He snapped them up, "zap, zap".

Then he looked for a safe hiding place. He found a spot under some rocks. He was so tired, that as soon as he put his head down, he fell fast asleep.

The green frog stayed in his hiding place until at last the rain came. First it came in a thin drizzle, "drip, drip". Then, it poured down, "'Swooosh, swooosh".

There was so much rain now that the frog thought it was a good idea to go back to his pond. This time he wasn't scared to hop through the garden. He knew now that if he went slowly and carefully, he would be safe.

When he reached his pond, it was full of water, and the water lilies showed off their big, pink flowers.

"Crack", "crack," he croaked happily as he hopped into the water. The sun came out, the insects returned, and he ate and ate. He wasn't hungry any longer, and he wasn't scared ever again.

Rob the Wombat

Rob was a brown wombat, strong and muscular with a body like a barrel. He lived deep in a forest in Tasmania. Visitors to Australia, who had never seen a wombat scurrying along looking for food before, thought he might be a badger.

When Rob was two years old, he no longer needed to stay with his mother for protection, or for food. He was ready to make his own burrow underground. Near the riverbank where grasses, moss, and the roots he liked to eat grew, he found just the right spot for his burrow. At first, heavy rain stopped him from digging. But, when the summer sun came out, it baked the ground until it was just right – not too hard nor too soft.

Rob dug and dug with his front paws until he had a long and wide burrow. Then he made a special place to sleep and lined it with tree bark and dried leaves. The burrow was deep enough to keep him cool in the heat of summer and warm in winter. Being underground, it protected him from eagles and foxes that ate wombats.

Rob wanted a front and back door to his burrow. As he was shy and preferred to live alone, he made certain that his burrow was not connected to the large colony of wombats on the hillside.

He liked his new home and felt so safe there that he slept most of the day, lying on his back and snoring softly. He grew fat and his coat grew shiny.

When the winds brought the winter, roots and grasses were hard to find. The cold weather kept him inside his burrow, and for the first time he was lonely.

When Rob's mother came to visit, she noticed that he looked sad. 'You are a silly wombat, Rob. It's nice to have friends popping in now and again.'

Rob scratched his furry head. 'Yes, it would be nice to have friends some of the time. Perhaps I could make my burrow longer and link it to the others on the hill, but it will be hard work.'

He thought about it and then went outside to check the ground. He would have to dig around a tree, and there would be roots he would have to chew through. But, he was sure that he could do it. He forgot his shyness and began to dig and dig. Each day his claws and sharp teeth cut through the roots.

Within a short while, he was close to the burrows of wombats on the hillside. They could hear him digging towards them. Wombats are not very friendly and don't like strangers. But, when Rob reached their burrows, they saw his muddy coat and dirty claws and felt sorry for him. They licked him clean and fed him the sweet grasses they had saved from summer.

Rob was very tired and fell asleep as soon as he closed his eyes. When he woke, at first he didn't know where he was, but then he remembered his long journey. After he had rested, he thanked the other wombats and went back to his burrow. Then he made a door into the long tunnel so that he could visit the wombats, or go back to his own home.

He visited the wombats on the hillside often. And one day he invited them all to his burrow. After their long underground journey, he welcomed them. He fed his visitors special roots and delicious, dried herbs he had stored. They all had a good meal.

Rob was happy and had lost his shyness. Now he had a very long burrow and friends on the hillside too. What more could a wombat want.

The Shy Wind

At the end of summer the Wind Family blew hard and strong. At that time of year their job was to cool the earth to prepare for winter, and spread seeds so that more plants and trees could grow. Only the youngest member of the family, six year old Jamie, refused to fill his chest and blow. Jamie was shy, and hid behind the clouds.

'I don't want to learn to blow,' Jamie said. 'I want to play here in the sky with my dog Gusty.' Jamie loved Gusty, a dog with tiny wings who was born in the wind.

Jamie's family was so busy blowing that they let him play in the clouds with Gusty.

One day, the Wind Family brought a huge storm. A gale howled and swirled as it swept across the black and purple sky. Jamie and Gusty were scared and clung together until all was quiet again.

After the gale, the sky was dotted with leaves, dirt and odd belongings from Earth like papers, shoes, socks and toys. The clouds complained loudly about the mess. The Wind Family promised to blow the sky clear again as soon as they had the time.

The Wind Nest in the clouds was meant to be a resting place, but now it was a mess. Jamie looked through all the things that had blown into the nest. He picked out a cuddly bear, a hat and a small, black hard thing that talked to him and made music, if he turned the knobs.

'What is it?' Jamie asked one of his sisters who was sweeping the nest.

'It's a radio, silly!' she puffed. 'Earthlings listen to it. Throw it away!'

Jamie liked the voices and music. Gusty liked the songs so much that he howled in tune to them.

'Wooooosss sstoppppitchugg,' his family blasted at Jamie in disgust. Throw that thing away. You're wasting your time with it. You're not like anyone in the Wind Family at all.'

'Woossstttttsu…tsu…tsuuuu,' Jamie wailed, and hid under a cloud.

'Let him have the silly thing for one more season…he's only little once,' his one grandmother puffed gently, and gave Jamie a hug. His other grandmother nodded in agreement.

'He's shy, but he'll grow up soon, and learn to do his job like all the other Wind Children,' his mother said blowing Jamie a kiss.

Autumn arrived, and the wind blew harder and sharper. People on earth shivered and drew their clothing tightly around their bodies. Their hair stood up or swept their faces, and they complained. It bent unhappy trees to breaking point, and their leaves fell in heaps on the ground. But, after school, children's kites flew higher and higher in the sky.

While most of Jamie's family went away on wind patrol, he decided it was time he learned to blow. So, he practised breathing in, expanding his chest and puffing out wind every day.

Jamie was listening to his radio, when he heard that a yacht was struggling to sail on a calm sea. The sailors were desperate as there hadn't been any wind to fill their sails for days.

Jamie knew that the yacht was only a short blow away, and he decided to try and help. 'I hope that I can make a wind strong enough to help the boat to sail,' he told Gusty.

With Gusty's help, he found the yacht quickly and filled his chest. He blasted again and again with all his strength. Ripples appeared in the sea and the yacht's sails fluttered in the breeze. Slowly it began to move. Just as Jamie was becoming tired of blowing, two of his older cousins arrived to help. Together they formed a team, and soon the yacht was well on its way.

When the Wind Family returned from patrolling the skies, they learned about Jamie's caring and bravery and were overcome with joy. Jamie was a hero and an example to his brothers and sisters.

'Woooooooo wooooooooo!' they blew loudly and proudly swirled around him.

The Trouble with Charlotte

Charlotte was a four year old beauty with shiny blue eyes and blonde hair. She was loved by her parents and two older sisters, but she was not happy. She worried constantly about being parted from her mother. She was scared that something awful would happen to her while her mother was away. Or, that her mother might get sick and die, like her friend Alice's mother, who died a few months earlier. She was upset if she was left with a minder, or even if her mother went outdoors to the post box. In the mornings when her mother dropped her off at kindergarten, she sobbed.

For Charlotte's birthday, her parents bought her a huge doll with blonde, curly hair like her own. Charlotte called the doll Evie and it became her special friend. She took Evie with her wherever she went. Evie even slept on her pillow. When Evie was with her, Charlotte wasn't as scared of being parted from her mother.

One Sunday morning during summer, the family went for a walk along the nearby lake. Of course Charlotte took Evie along. They were all enjoying the walk when Charlotte slipped. She was unhurt apart from a grazed knee, but Evie flew out of her arms and landed in mud. When her dad picked up her doll, it was covered in thick mud. Charlotte sobbed. Her mother and sisters tried to calm her but, nothing helped.

Charlotte's sister Nadine, who was good at sewing and painting, hugged Charlotte. 'Don't cry Lottie. I promise to fix Evie, and you'll have her to love again.'

'But she'll never be the same. She's such a mess.'

Nadine kissed her little sister. 'I promise that I'll work on her until she's like new.'

At home, Nadine put the doll in the sun to dry, and then shook it hard to get rid of most of the mud. Every day after school she worked on the doll. She removed the dirty clothes, washed them gently and dried them. Then she cleaned the little body. Fortunately Evie wasn't scratched or broken, but her golden hair was filthy. Carefully Nadine removed the doll's wig. She washed each strand of hair and made tiny curls. Soon the doll had a head of bouncy curls. As the dress was torn in a few places, Nadine repaired it with lace and ribbons. She made a pair of new white socks for Evie to go with her tiny polished shoes. When the doll was almost ready to return to Charlotte, she made a little crown for her head.

At first, Charlotte was lost without Evie. Her grazed knee healed, and while Nadine was repairing her doll, she became used to being without her. She was growing up and stopped crying when her mother left her at kindergarten in the morning. She no longer worried that bad things would happen.

One day, when Charlotte returned from kindergarten, Nadine surprised her. Evie was sitting on her bed. At first Charlotte stared at Evie without saying a word. Then, she inspected the doll and gave Evie's little face a kiss.

'You look like a princess now, Evie,' she whispered to the doll. Charlotte ran to find her sister to give her a "thank you" hug and a big kiss.

The girls' thrilled mother praised Nadine's hard work. She turned to Charlotte and said, 'You see my darling, some things can be fixed... they can be even better than they were before. Never ever give up!'

Charlotte nodded thoughtfully. 'Evie is looking so beautiful now that I think she should stay on the chair in my room most of the time. I don't think I should carry her about with me anymore.'

For Older Children & Preteens

Ava's Computer

Ten-year-old Ava's King Charles Cavalier Spaniel, was called Brandy. He slept at the bottom her bed at night, waiting for her to come home after school, and sat at her feet when she was working on her computer. He went to Ava's older sister, Ella and her younger brother, James too, but only for short periods.

Once Ava had completed her homework, she groomed Brandy and played ball with him. Unlike many of her class mates, in the time left until dinner she didn't chat with her friends on Facebook or play computer games. She searched for information online. If she learned something new or interesting at school, she would "google" it when she came home to find out more. Her interest was animals, especially dogs. She made certain that Brandy was receiving the best food for his age. Once she learned that Spaniels often had ear problems, she cleaned his droopy ears each time she groomed him.

Brandy grew into a magnificent dog. When Ava took him to the park for a run people stopped to admire him. He learned new words and listened to Ava's commands of "sit", "stay" or "go". When Brandy looked at her with his large, brown eyes she knew he understood.

Ava tickled Brandy's tummy. 'My clever boy!' she said to him. 'Dogs are so interesting…pack animals, and yet dogs like you are our best friends.' His shiny eyes and wagging tail at the sound of her voice was all she needed in reply.

One evening, when dinner was almost ready, Ava's Mum found her at the computer with Brandy asleep at her feet.

'You're back at the computer again. It's not good for you to be hooked on it, Ava. Don't you want to unwind a bit? You could spend some time with Ella and James.'

'I'm discovering new things Mum, it's important,' Ava replied.

'Learning is good ... as long as you're enjoying it, my darling.'

'Thanks Mum.'

Ava whispered to Brandy, 'There's no time to explain to Mum yet that I'm learning about dogs…but I will one day.'

During school holidays the family went to the beach. They took their caravan and an extra tent. As Brandy was a timid dog, Ava worried about taking him with them. She told her Dad that she thought it best to leave him with their next door neighbour who owned a Spaniel too. As Brandy often played with the neighbour's dog, she thought he would be happier there.

They all enjoyed their holiday. The days were warm and the sea was calm enough for swimming. Ava's Dad and James went fishing most days, while Ava, Ella and Mum walked on the beach, collected shells, and talked to people they met along the way. The girls helped with cooking on the barbeque, and James and Dad cleaned up.

One night, just before bed, a large black dog wandered into their tent.

'I haven't seen that dog around before,' Emma said.

'She might be hungry, I'll give her some leftover meat,' James said.

'No wait James. Stay where you are!' Ava said with an authority in her voice that her family were not used to hearing.

Ava looked at the dog carefully. It was female. She remembered reading about signs of aggression in bitches. The dog's tail was straight, her eyes were staring and she was growling. At any moment she could attack.

'Keep away from the dog everyone!' Ava's Dad said, looking worried.

Don't worry Dad. I know what to do. I've read a lot about angry, aggressive dogs. I'll distract her while the rest of you move slowly out of the tent into the caravan,' Ava said.

'Ava! Be careful,' her mother added worriedly.

'Go when I give you the word! I know what to do,' Ava said, her voice strong and confident.

Meanwhile, Ava had been forming a ball in her hand from the shiny, left over tinfoil they had used to cook their meat.

'Go now!' Ava, as she held the tinfoil ball up so the dog could see it. Then she threw it out of the tent. The dog followed the ball smelling of meat. Quickly, Ava closed the tent flap and ran through to the caravan.

'Phew that was a close call,' Ava said. 'The tent flap is closed now. I don't think she'll bother us anymore. But I guess you'd better check, James.'

'She's gone,' James said with relief.

Ava's parents took their turns in hugging Ava, and telling her how brave she was.

'Just as well you insisted on not bringing Brandy along,' her Dad said.

'That stray might've had a go at him. Better not think of what could've happened,' Emma said.

Ava nodded.

'You were amazing,' James said. 'Wonder Woman! I can't wait to tell my friends at school about my brave sister.'

Ella hugged Ava. 'Thank you! I'm the older sister, but I didn't have a clue what to do…none of us did except you. How did you know?'

'I've been doing some reading about dogs on the Internet, trying to find out as much as I can about them. I read about aggressive bitches on heat…and recognised the signs. It's nothing special.'

'Oh yes it is,' Ava's Mum said as she handed Ava a hot cup of cocoa. 'I was silly to try to stop you learning all you can. You're like your Dad who enjoys studying. I am going to do a bit more study too. I think we all should.'

Ava took her mother's hand, and lovingly squeezed it.

Goldie and Me

At last, after two years of pleading, I was in the pet shop with Mum, Dad and my sister Zoe, looking at the puppies for sale.

'I know that you haven't been happy at school lately, Sam. Maybe having a puppy will help,' Mum said gently.

I knew immediately which puppy I wanted. I pointed to the smallest one in the litter. 'She's the one I want.'

'She's very small, but it's your choice,' Dad said.

Mum preferred one of the bigger puppies clawing at the cage. 'He looks active and healthy.'

'No, I want her!' I said, raising my voice.

'I think she's very cute,' Zoe said.

I was surprised that my sister agreed with me. She didn't always.

The woman who owned the pet shop lifted the puppy out of the cage, then handed her to me. 'Hold her for a while and then make up your mind.'

'Do you think she's the best choice?' Dad asked.

'The best choice is the one your son wants,' the woman replied. 'She's a good natured, healthy dog. She'll gain weight soon.'

'Please Dad, I want her.' I said, stroking the puppy's head.

'That's it then. She's yours, Sam,' Mum said. 'But you'll have to feed her and train her not to mess.'

'Yes, Mum. I will, I promise.'

The woman smiled warmly at me. She handed me a list of feeding instructions and placed a hand on my shoulder. 'If you have any questions about your puppy I'll try to help.'

We left the pet shop with the puppy, a basket, and bag of puppy food.

When we arrived home I let the puppy wander. She wanted to smell the chairs, the legs of the tables, the carpet and everything else. Then I took her into the back garden. 'This is where you'll play during the day,' I said to her.

She looked at me and for the first time she wagged her tail. I gave her a bowl of food. She emptied it quickly and then jumped into my arms.

'You know you're mine,' I said to her softly.

'What are you going to call her,' Zoe asked.

'Goldie. She's such a lovely golden colour.'

'Yes, the name suits her.'

I smiled and sighed a happy sigh. All my nagging had been worthwhile.

The puppy fell asleep, and I placed her in her basket.

'You'll be a strong dog one day,' I said to her, giving her a pat. I tiptoed away.

Near the door I passed the mirror. I saw the reflection of my small, thin body. *I wish I could grow bigger and stronger, so that the others in class would stop laughing at me and calling me nasty names.*

Goldie learned quickly. 'You're doing a good job with training your puppy. I'm proud of you,' Mum said, looking happy.

'I think Goldie should go to puppy school,' Dad added.

I giggled and said, 'I didn't know that puppies went to school too.'

On the next Saturday, we took Goldie to puppy school. There were lots of puppies and their owners there. When Goldie saw the other dogs she trembled, hid between my legs refusing to move.

The instructor came to talk to us. 'Your puppy is nervous. She will have to be socialised before she can learn instructions,' he said.

'Socialised? What does he mean?' I asked Dad.

'She has to learn to get along with other dogs before she can learn instructions at puppy school,' he said.

On the way back home I stroked Goldie. I worried about her all weekend. I knew what it was like to be scared. Then, Mum had a good idea. 'Let's ask the woman at the pet shop what to do.'

The next day after school, we went to the pet shop, and I told the lady how scared Goldie was.

'She's big enough now for a collar and a lead. Take her down to the park on a lead. There are other dogs there. Slowly let her get used to them.'

'Thank you, that's a good idea,' I said.

'But remember not to hurry her.'

Goldie didn't like her collar at first, but she got used it. Then I clipped the lead onto her collar so that we could practise walking around the garden.

A few days later, Mum drove us to the park. Goldie's lead was on, and I opened the car door. She left the car slowly and sniffed the grass. Her ears were up as she listened to the other dogs. At least she didn't run back to the car.

The park was three blocks from our house, close enough to walk there. Soon she got used to the other dogs and wagged her tail when I took out her lead. I was nervous at the park too. I kept my head down at first, and avoided talking to any of the dog owners or other children, but after a while I recognised people who were there every day. Soon I was saying "hello", and smiling back when they greeted me. Other children brought their dogs to the park and we walked our dogs together.

Goldie had learned to "come" when I called her. I was teaching her to obey simple commands so well that Dad said she didn't need to go to puppy school. I took Goldie for long walks too. Sometimes we went to the shops or past my school.

She was growing into a strong, big dog. The muscles in my legs were growing bigger too from such a lot of walking. Some other things changed as well. I was so used to talking to people at the park that at school I had almost forgotten how nasty my classmates had been to me. The first time I greeted them, they stared at me surprised. They stopped being horrid to me, but they didn't ask me to play games with them. I made a new friend, Simon. He had a dog and a cat, so we sat together with a lot to chat about over recess.

One morning, Zoe left the side gate open. Goldie ran out, all the way to the school to look for me. When school was out I saw a crowd of children gathered around her. As soon as she saw me, she ran to me.

'You have a beautiful dog,' one of the boys said.

'Yes, I love her,' I replied proudly.

They wanted to know her name and asked all about her.

Goldie brought me luck. During recess the next day, the boys in the class said I could play ball with them. I told them I would only play with them if Simon played as well. When they agreed we both joined in the game. I surprised them by running fast and jumping high to catch the ball. Simon was not much good at ball games, but they did not pick on him.

Months later, I was walking to my classroom when I heard someone behind the stairs crying. It was Dan, one of the boys who had been mean to me. When he saw me he turned away and tried to dry his eyes with his sleeve. At first I felt like walking away from him, but I didn't.

'What's up Dan?' I asked.

He started to cry again.

'Come on.'

'It's my dog, Rover. He's sick…I'm scared he'll die. My Dad says the vet is too expensive.'

'Oh that's sad. I would cry too if Goldie was sick.'

'I wanted to stay at home today to look after him, but Mum made me come to school,' Dan said.

'I think I know someone who might be able to help.'

'Really?' He looked up for the first time.

I told him about the kind lady at the pet shop who knew a lot about dogs.

'Maybe she can help Rover.'

I arranged to meet Dan at the pet shop that afternoon. The owner was busy with customers and we waited until she came up to us. 'I see you've brought your friend today. How can I help?'

Dan told her about his sick dog. She listened and then asked him lots of questions. 'Your dog should definitely see a vet, but you could try to give him some of this first.' She handed him a bottle. 'It won't harm him…and it could help.'

Dan put his hand in a pocket. He pulled out three gold coins. 'I haven't much money, but I can pay the rest later.'

'No charge today. Just come past and tell me how your dog is doing,' the lady said.

I saw Dan at school, but I didn't want to ask how Rover was in case the medicine had made him worse.

One morning, Dan was waiting for me. 'I've got wonderful news. Rover is as good as new … and it's thanks to you.'

'That's good, Dan. I'm pleased.'

'Will you come round to my house one afternoon to play with Rover? She's good with other dogs, so you can bring Goldie along too.'

A year later, Goldie had grown into a beautiful, strong dog. I was still thin, but I was taller and much happier. Mum said that I'd had a "growth spurt". I loved Goldie and I knew that my life had changed because of her.

Loren and the Orange Cat

Ten year old Loren felt lonely and sad most of the time, but no one noticed. Her brother Gary was fifteen and ignored her. He hung out with his friends, was home in time for diner, but then disappeared into his room. Loren's father died just before she was born and her Mum worked long hours. After work she was tired, ate her evening meal and fell into bed.

Most weekends, Loren helped her Mum to clean the apartment and prepare meals for the week ahead. Once the chores were completed, her mother usually slept to recover from the week's work. They hardly went out apart from an occasional movie, or for a hurried meal at MacDonald's. No one ever visited.

From time to time her mother asked, 'Is everything going well at school?'

Loren would nod.

Then, her Mum usually said, 'If anything is upsetting you, tell me about it and I will try to help.'

One look at her mother's tired face told Loren that it was best not to bother her with any of her own worries.

Loren had pretty features, but her long black hair worn pulled back in a ponytail didn't flatter her. When she looked in the mirror, she hated her image. *I'm ugly, no wonder the bullies call me "fatty" and "pig face"*. She felt safest at home where she could not be seen by others.

Fortunately, her school was only two blocks from home. She could walk to school quickly, looking ahead without stopping until she reached the school gate. Inside school, she kept her head down, avoiding the bullies with their loud voices and nasty comments. Loren and her two shy friends stuck together to stay safe.

Loren's grandmother waited for her after school every day. Though Loren loved her grandmother, once they had eaten, they hardly talked. Gran, as Loren called her, was almost deaf. She spent the afternoon in a comfortable armchair knitting in front of the television turned up high. The noise of the television blasted into every corner of the small apartment. When at last the old woman turned off the television for a snooze, things did not improve much, as she snored loudly. Cotton wool in her ears didn't help Loren, but some special jelly ear buds she found in the bathroom cabinet fitted so well that they almost drowned the noise.

There were no children Loren's age in the small apartment building, and her two school friends lived far away. After doing her homework, Loren played with a cat that belonged to Mrs. Dubinsky, two doors away. The large cat called Sweetie was as fat as his owner, and they both had orange hair. As overfed as the cat was, he didn't refuse an offering of some meat or fish Loren saved for him. Mrs. Dubinsky kept Sweetie inside the apartment. When Loren visited, the old woman stood by the door careful not to let her cat escape. The heavy traffic close to the apartment had killed her last cat, and she wasn't going to let it happen again.

The block of apartments overlooked a park. Each day, Loren stared out at the park from the window in her bedroom, watched the trees change with the seasons, the flowers bloom, and the children playing. She longed to go to the park, but the thought of people seeing her ugly body, or meeting up with the school bullies scared her. Once her grandma had settled in her chair, Loren knew that there was no point in asking her to come with her to the park.

One afternoon, Loren was looking through the window at trees in the park swaying in the wind, when she saw Sweetie run across the grass towards a tall tree. She had seen a terrified cat stuck high in a tree, and when Sweetie began to climb the tree, she worried.

The park was quiet at that time of day, and no one seemed to have noticed the cat in the tree. Without a thought, Loren ran out of the building into the park. The tree was easy to find, but she couldn't see Sweetie amongst the foliage. When she spotted him, she called him, but he ignored her and climbed to a higher branch. Loren waited patiently for Sweetie to become tired, or hungry enough to come down. An hour must have passed, when she heard the calls of her grandmother and Mrs. Dubinsky. The two old women had hobbled into the park looking for her and the cat. When Sweetie heard his owner telling him to come down, he attempted to climb down to a lower branch, but could not climb backwards. Poor Sweetie was stuck. First he meowed, then he yoweled. Curiosity had made him climb up, but fear wouldn't let him come down. Loren had not climbed a tree before and stood there helplessly.

A crowd gathered, and children stared at the stuck orange cat. Everyone was talking about how to rescue Sweetie when one of the boys climbed up to the branch where Sweetie was stuck. He must've known a lot about cats because he talked to him softly, then he grabbed him. A friend at the bottom of the tree climbed up half way, and together they managed to bring him down.

When Loren's mother heard about Sweetie's rescue and Loren's first visit to the park, she was shocked. 'I had no idea you were afraid of going to the park. I thought you played there every afternoon and didn't even ask, but I should've. I've been too caught up with work and poor Gran is too old to spend time with you.'

Loren tried her best to reassure her mother, as she usually did, but when her mother put her arms around her and kissed her, she burst into tears.

'I'm ugly and fat, no one likes me…and I get bullied,' she blurted out. 'That's why I don't go to the park.'

'My poor darling! You're just a little overweight, but it's natural "puppy fat", and you'll lose it soon. You're definitely not ugly. It's your hair that doesn't suit you, my darling.'

Loren burst into tears again.

'Let's go into the bathroom and we'll do something different with your hair.'

Loren sat in front of the mirror, while her mother removed the rubber band from her pony tail. She brushed Loren's hair and brought it forward around her face. 'See how it suits you. How about going to my hairdresser for a cut and blow dry? You won't believe the change it will make.'

The next day Loren nervously arrived at the hairdresser.

'Don't worry Honey, I'm going to make you look pretty.'

As the hairdresser began to cut her hair, Loren closed her eyes. When she opened them, she had a soft bob that completely changed her appearance.

'Oh…is that really me?' she said.

'It certainly is. You have a lovely face and this style suits you. I will show you how to look after it so that it looks good every day. And when your hair grows again you can come back for another cut.'

When Loren arrived home, her brother whistled and her grandmother gave her a hug.

'You look lovely, my darling,' her mother said, and kissed her. 'I told you that you would.'

Loren noticed a change in herself. It wasn't only her hair. She felt a little more confident. She held her head high as she walked through the school gates the next day. Girls in her class gathered around her complementing her on her new hairstyle. Some asked for the name of her hairdresser. No one called her names again or mentioned her weight. She even walked past the park after school. Children she had talked to when Sweetie was stuck saw her and waved to her, but she still felt too unsure of herself to join them.

That night while preparing dinner, her mother talked to her. 'Things have to change for both of us. I talked to my boss and guess what? He said he'd noticed how tired I was looking. From now on I will have two afternoons off work every week. He will pay me more for the hours I work, so I won't lose any money. We can go out and spend more time together. We can go to the park or wherever you like.'

Loren gave her mother a hug. Then she went to the fridge, cut a soft piece of fish and rolled it into tin foil. It was a special treat for Sweetie.

The Outsider

Eleven-year old Tarek was a new student at a school in the Eastern suburbs of Melbourne. He looked like the other students in a pre-worn blazer from the school's charity shop. Even his underwear had been handed down from his brothers and cousins. When he received the blazer, he brushed it and held it to his body until the smell of the previous owner was gone. His class teacher welcomed him and explained to the class that he was from Iraq. Two boys volunteered to be "buddies" to help Tarek settle into the school. Though they tried to be helpful and friendly, he made it clear to them that he did not want assistance. All that concerned him was learning. He sat in the front of the class and focused on the lesson. The social activities the school offered didn't interest him.

Tarek was so tall for his age that he could've played for the school's basketball team, but he was not interested in sport. He had made only one friend at school, Rashid who was one class above him, and didn't play sport either. Before school and during recess the two boys hung out in corners of the playground and didn't mix with the other students. Even Rashid knew little about Tarek's background, other than that he and his family were refugees from Iraq who had arrived in Australia two years earlier. Every time Rashid asked a question about Tarek's past, or about Iraq he was met with a silent stare. Though skinny, Tarek was far too tall and muscular for any of the bullies to make a move on him. His dark eyes glared fiercely with such intense focus, and he cursed them so loudly that no one dared confront him. None of the students could've known that he felt afraid and uncertain at the new school. Though he was grateful to have found a place of safety in Australia, it was different from anything he knew, and each day was a challenge. He was more accustomed to a larger class where a teacher wrote on the blackboard. In his new school, the class was smaller, and the style of teaching was different. Pupils were encouraged to ask questions and make suggestions during the lesson.

He barely talked to the other students in his classes, though he had mastered sufficient English to read, write and speak the language. He was particularly good at math, and every day his homework was completed without errors. If he had been more talkative in class his teachers would've found him an ideal pupil. Eventually class members gave up trying to communicate with him and ignored him. At the end of his first year at the school, he passed all his exams with high grades.

He remained reticent, and would've been almost invisible if not for an incident in the third week of the term. Though it was a cold day, most of the students wanted to be outdoors during the break. The teachers were involved in a meeting in the staff room, at the far end of the school.

While Tarek ate his lunch, he watched a tight group of the youngest boys talking and laughing. When he saw a fine spiral of smoke, he stood. The group of boys had ignored school rules and had lit a small fire with bits of wood to warm their hands. A sudden scream from one of the boys was followed by rising flames. Tarek rushed towards the fire, where a ring of students had gathered.

In his loudest voice he took control, pushing students out the path of the fire and barking instructions. 'Everyone move away from the flames.' He pointed to one of the boys. 'You, run to the staff room as fast as you can…tell the teachers about the fire… and to call the fire brigade.'

He noticed that young Jeremy's jumper had caught alight. Quickly, he threw off his blazer, grabbed Jeremy and rolled him in it until the flames were staunched. Still using his blazer, he beat the flames. 'Come on, you others, help me!' he shouted.

By the time the time teachers arrived most of the flames were extinguished. At last the fire brigade and an ambulance came. The firemen used their hoses to douse remaining flames and embers still flickering. Jeremy had some nasty burns and was taken to hospital by ambulance.

Once the emergency was over, the principal called a meeting of students, teachers, as well as worried parents who had heard about the fire, and had come to the school He talked about the incident in detail and about the dangers of lighting fires. In strong tones, he stated that in future anyone attempting to light a fire on school grounds would be expelled.

Then the principal's voice softened. 'We have someone here to thank for his immediate and clear-headed action that not only probably saved Jeremy from extensive burns, but prevented a huge fire from taking hold and even burning down our school. His name is Tarek. Please stand Tarek, so that people can see you.'

Everyone craned their necks to see the hero, but Tarek embarrassed by the attention, tried to ignore the call. When the students began to clap loudly and call out, 'Ta…rek, Ta…rek, Ta…rek,' he was forced to stand. More clapping and stamping followed.

The next day, none of the students wanted to do their school work. They gathered around Tarek asking questions.

The teacher called out, 'Everyone back in their seats, please.' Turning to Tarek, she spoke gently, searching for the right words. 'Tarek, you have been very quiet since joining us. If you would like to tell us about yourself we would all be very interested, and happy to hear it.'

The children clapped and waited.

Tarek stood slowly. 'I have a very long story…and I don't know where to start but I will try my best.'

Slowly and tentatively he told the class that he was born on a farm in a small village about sixty kilometres from Baghdad.

'It is a beautiful village in the hills near a river. My grandfather grew wheat and rice and we lived with him in his house.' His eyes misted and he swallowed. 'We kept goats, sheep and we had dogs. I owned a cat and I loved her so much. I gave her an American name, Rocket because she ran fast.'

He told the class that his father was an engineer who worked in the city. Then he talked about his two older brothers. One was an engineer too, and the other was studying computers at university. His younger brother and a sister were at school.

Talking about his family was overwhelming, and he was unable to continue. He sat with his head on the desk cradled in his arms.

The teacher touched him gently and handed him a glass of water. 'It's ok to be upset Tarek.'

She stood at the front of the class. 'Carry on with the exercise we were meant to do today, class. Tarek will talk to us again when he is ready.'

A while later Tarek asked if he could go home. He didn't return to school for the rest of that week, but on the following Monday he greeted class members, something he had not done before. After a short discussion with the teacher he continued with his story.

He explained that talking about his home brought back painful memories he tried to forget. His hands were clenched and his face pale, as he explained how Al Queda had attacked and set fire to many of the houses in his village, including his own. The class listened as he told them that when he was four years old his mother was murdered by Al Queda, part of his village burned, and their livestock killed.

'That is how I learned how to put out a fire and try to save lives,' he said with a sigh.

His father was at work, and with no one home to care for him or his younger brother and sister, they went to live with their aunt in a neighbouring village. The attacks were constant, and as it became increasingly dangerous for them to take the bus to Baghdad they remained at home, and were taught by his aunt. He smiled for the first time, remembering how knowledgeable but strict she was.

Around this time, his father called the family together to tell them that as their lives were at risk, he had made an application to emigrate to Australia, and that they were accepted. They would leave within a year. Australia seemed so far away, but everyone realised their father was right, and that they had to seek a safer place to live. 'We will all speak English now and not a word of Arabic. We must learn to speak their language before we leave,' their father said sternly.

By now, Tarek's speech was halting, and he became tearful as he tried to describe the flight from Baghdad and his arrival in Melbourne. He began to say how grateful he felt when he landed on Australian soil, but was overcome with emotion. The teacher suggested he stop and continue his story another day. He nodded gratefully, but before stopping he added with a choked voice, 'The people here were so kind…they helped us to find a home and work for my father…but I do still miss my home.'

The teacher thanked Tarek for telling the class his story. Then looking serious she added, 'If Tarek hadn't become our hero putting out the fire, we wouldn't have known about him or his terrible difficulties in Iraq, or how much he misses home. This is a lesson for all of us to be more tolerant of new or different people and to help them settle. Migrants from other countries bring their own special story - their experiences, culture and their unique abilities, and they enrich our country.'

The room was still after she finished speaking. Then mutters of agreement could be heard throughout the class.

Mindfulness

In the Fast Lane

I was twenty-one when I started working as a copy writer at a slick advertising agency. All my friends thought I had a perfect job surrounded by people with amazing ideas. The best part they thought, was that we started around 10:00 p.m., but they forgot about the long hours we worked at night.

There are perks in agencies. We had a spacious, stylishly decorated office. There were some fun things like a pool table and a place for dogs if people wanted to bring them to work. Most Fridays, we had parties with free wine, beer and snacks. In summer we fired up the *barbie* on the large balcony. We played hard, but no one lasts at an advertising agency unless they work hard too.

Being creative and unconventional was an important part of the work image that some people exploited in the way they dressed. Marvin, a graphic artist, who had the desk next to me made a point of looking like a Victorian gentleman. Rachel wore bright, long skirts and Hippie flowers in her hair. Others sported their tattoos and weird hairdos. But, the people who handled client's accounts dressed conservatively. Dressing up to create an image was not for me. I had too much on my mind creating the concepts of our advertisements to bother.

On the down side, we had deadlines, and we drank strong coffee late into the night to keep going. There was enormous competition between staff, and there were office politics as in most places. To keep up with the high pressure, some people used drugs on a regular basis. Most days I was high enough without any drugs.

Apart from initial ideas, just about everything was created technologically in high definition. It was fun. I loved the glossy images, the hype, clichés and smart copy. I was driven, working on several accounts at once, lost in my head, planning new smart lines. Naturally my bosses didn't complain. They were getting more than their money's worth from me.

Travelling to and from work was easiest by train. If seats were available, I read my emails, logged onto Facebook and Twitter to keep up with the latest happenings, and my online buddies. Once I was home, the television was on to watch out for latest news headlines, and my laptop and phone were next to me. With so much happening a relationship was out of the question, and during the week I rarely went out. Eating was something I did while on line.

Food from the deli or the supermarket heated in the microwave and a few glasses of wine were all I needed, or so I thought. There was so much to keep me involved on the Internet, from games I was hooked on, to fun gambling. With all this stimulation, I could not switch off to sleep, and went to bed late, taking my phone with me to check the last messages of the day. I was beyond tired, but I did not listen to my body crying out to me to slow down.

I had become a techno addict and I enjoyed it all until eventually it got to me. At work I began to sneak quick checks for text messages on my phone, and went to the toilet to answer messages from my Facebook friends. My concentration on my work slipped. My light quirky adverts that the clients liked, were now heavy and boring. My team and the bosses noticed and commented, but hoped that I was merely going through a phase that would change soon.

Around this time, I came down with a nasty bug. I phoned the office and stayed in bed. My head ached too much for any noise. Concentration on my laptop was out. I hadn't spent time alone in my apartment without all my electronic stuff turned on since I'd moved in sixteen months earlier. Within two days, I was sleeping more and waking early enough to hear choruses of birds. I was dizzy and weak, but I made it to the kitchen. I had my toast and tea on my small balcony. I had not been out there for so long that I'd forgotten how delightfully sunny it was. I noticed how much the pot plants I had planted when I moved in had grown and were flowering, though I hadn't watered them.

Relaxing felt strange at first, but pleasant. As my strength returned, I took long walks and ate at places I hadn't been to before. This slower way of life was appealing, but I knew it was temporary. I enjoyed my work, but I knew that I would have to make some changes. Right then I had no idea what changes to make.

When I returned to work eight days later, a promotion of boxed CD's about mindful meditation was a new project waiting for me. The idea of mindfulness or "living in the moment" was something I had often joked about. But, after listening to one of the CD's I was impressed. It made me aware of an alternative way of living. Curious about the new ideas, I listened again and again. There *was* a way to "go easier on myself". With a new clarity I saw how I was driving myself, not eating correctly or exercising. I was a one dimensional creature obsessed by work and technology. I don't believe in coincidences - this project had turned up at a time when I needed it most.

I liked the idea of mediating daily, but being a realistic person, I knew that my life was too busy to promise myself that I would, or could, stick to it on a regular basis. It would be useful to help me control those panicky moments when I felt as if I was falling apart.

Recently, I've been slowing down enough to be aware of the sunset, an enjoyable conversation, or a tasty meal, and I sleep more. My creativity has been given a boost, but in a less driven way. I am more directed, waste less time, and leave work earlier. The quality of my work has improved with fresher ideas. Clients have noticed, and my bosses have noticed too. I am enjoying work in a less frenetic way and occasionally I go out during the week. Preventing myself from being caught up with excessive technology at home has been important. As hard as it is, I turn off all the machines an hour before bed. I push myself out of the office for a short walk to buy fresh fruit and a healthy sandwich for lunch. I've met a few new people and I've begun to socialise more. Though I'm hoping for a serious relationship, so far it hasn't happened.

There are times when I slip back, but the main thing is that life is more fun. I'm enjoying being aware of the world around me instead of being constantly lost in my head.

Mindful Work

Jordan, an administrator in a government office, was making his way home after his day at work. It was the busiest time of year, his head ached, and his thoughts raced with the pressure of work. He had tried to complete the mountain of reports and the accounts for his section, but finishing it all it meant leaving out details, and he thought the details were important. He barely took breaks, and at one stage during the afternoon his eyes became misty, he went blank and slightly dizzy. He put his head down for a few minutes, had a strong coffee, and went back to work.

When he eventually left work, he almost missed his stop. As he walked the few blocks to his home, he did not notice the glorious new spring blossoms in the streets and gardens, and was barely aware of the drizzle. His thoughts were on the work he still had to catch up on at home. What if he could not manage to finish all he needed to before tomorrow, he worried. Once inside, he greeted his wife, threw off his damp coat, and joined the family at the dinner table. With his mind still on work, his wife Arlene's chatter and his children's news about school passed without his attention. After dinner, he attempted to catch up with his work on the computer, but within an hour his mind and body had other ideas. After an hour, he had passed out, his head on the desk. When he woke, the family was asleep, and the house was dark and quiet.

The next day, Jordan's boss, Reid walked past his desk. The two men had been to the same school and had been friends in their youth.

'Let's have a chat in my office,' Reid said.

Jordan rose from his seat.

He's sure to find errors, and be unhappy that I haven't been able to complete the set of figures.

'Good news Jordan, I'm getting you an assistant. There's far too much work for one person to cope with, though I know you're trying very hard…too hard. It's an impossible task. The business is expanding and doing well enough now…and we can afford it.'

Jordan nodded. 'I've tried my best but…'

'I know you always try hard…and you've been conscientious ever since we were kids at school, but life is to be lived. Put some energy into something outside of work that you enjoy.'

On the bus home, Reid's words echoed in Jordan's mind. *"Life is to be lived." Yes, Reid is right. He knows me well.*

He smiled at the person next to him and looked through the window at people rushing home. As he walked home from the bus stop, he noticed the blossoms for the first time.

That night, Jordan thought about Reid's comment again. *"Life is to be lived."* Of course Reid was right, but how could he become involved in something else when he had no hobbies? He wasn't aware of enjoying anything except his work, or being with his wife and children. His work had absorbed almost all his energy.

At least I can rest easy tonight and enjoy sleeping without worrying about work. Reid has opened a door for me. I can spend more time with Arlene and the children and enjoy some time for myself.

Reid kept his word and employed Pete as Jordan's assistant. The two men developed a friendly working relationship. Working at a steady pace with reasonable breaks, the piles of unattended material diminished. After work Jordan devoted more time to his wife and family, and they even took a short holiday together.

Over the next few weeks, Jordan remembered some of the activities he had enjoyed before he started working. At school he was excellent at carpentry. Later he'd enjoyed playing squash, hiking and debating. He knew he needed to be fitter and thought about going to a gym, but joining a debating group interested him most.

I'm a lucky man to be able to have a fuller and more meaningful life.

A Special Day

Rachel fumbled to still the shrieking alarm and hesitantly opened her eyes. A slight headache and foul taste remained from the wine she had drank the night before. A tense, uptight feeling was with her almost all the time. She worried about small things that seemed to matter, but they were soon replaced by new concerns.

She pulled back the blankets, yawned, and padded across the floor. A welcoming purr and furry tail wound around her legs. She bent to stroke the cat that had become a large part of her life. When her cat was purring on her lap she felt more relaxed.

Pools of gold poured into the kitchen, and she smiled her first relieved smile. She had the day off work. Being good at math had landed her a secure job in an accountant's office. The job turned out to be boring, but the money was good, the people she worked with were pleasant and she had some time off work, which was a big plus.

I'll have to think of finding more interesting work…that is if I am able to find another job in this tight market. Anyway, no time for worrying about that now…I'll have to hurry if I want to get to my painting group.

On her free morning, Rachel attended a small painting workshop with people who had become friends. She enjoyed attending the group, though the members had their different styles.

A quick shower, juice and a piece of toast is all I'll manage if I'm to make it.

She tried to avoid wasting time with her appearance, and dressed quickly in the jeans and tee shirt she had laid out the night before. If she avoided looking in the mirror she knew she would save time. Hurriedly, she flicked her fingers through her curls and applied a slick of lipstick. Before leaving, she grabbed a packet of biscuits from the pantry to share with her friends for morning tea. Then she checked and rechecked that the cat had sufficient food, and that all the appliances were turned off.

She placed the large painting she had worked on over the weekend against the car. She glanced at it, before going back to the house for her bag of paints and brushes. It wasn't her usual landscape or flowers, but an abstract with bold swirls of colour.

Perhaps they won't like it. Abstracts aren't always popular with the group…and possibly the brushwork is too free, the forms too dominant.

Before placing her painting in the boot, she noticed a sunny, shimmering haze of pink against the white wall of her house. The luscious, pink camellias were in full bloom with birds feeding on the nectar rich flowers. She stopped, stood still, and took a deep breath of the flowery perfume, as she admired the magnificent sight.

Seeing this glorious camellia bush today has been a gift. It's time I enjoyed the world around me…tried to stop listening to my scared voice. It prevents me from enjoying so much.

She put her painting in the boot, shutting it with a bang.

If only I'd use the advice in all the self-help books I read! I have to stop worrying…and learn to take fair criticism about my painting. And anyway, the more experienced artists in the group will probably be kind and help me to improve my technique. But, I do like the design and colours I've chosen in my painting, and no one will talk me out of it. I'm sticking to them.

The cool morning had a sharp edge. In the slow traffic, she noticed the mountains in the distance and the lush shrubs blooming in the gardens she passed.

What a lovely change from the closed dark city office and dreary work.

At the cemetery, there was a blocked line of traffic. Tractors and trucks halted the line of cars, safety beacons flashed, and road workers in fluorescent vests cautioned her to slow down. She allowed her worries about traffic slowing her down to float away. There was nothing she could do about it - she'd be late.

As she inched forward, she watched a woman clutching a bunch of flowers pass through the old cemetery gates. Young parents followed, urging two reluctant children through the grounds. As she waited, images of her departed loved ones formed a delicate kaleidoscope in her memory. Her father would be pleased that she was still painting, and had a steady job as well. He had said so many times that "most artists never ever made a living."

At last, moving traffic ended her reverie. She drove the rest of the way slowly. There was so much to be aware of during her drive. When she arrived at her destination, she unloaded her painting equipment.

I'm pleased I came today, even if I am a bit late. I'm going to enjoy painting, chatting with friends over the tea break, and sharing ideas about our work.

She enjoyed the workshop and smiled as she drove home.

They all liked my painting and were pleased that I was trying something new. They made a few suggestions too that I'll try tomorrow.

At home she was thoughtful.

I have this weekly window to the outside world, weekends to socialise, go for walks, or work on my painting. I can stay on in my secure job until I find more interesting work. It's time to stop drinking so much, in an attempt to blot out my worries.

I am fortunate.

A Lesson from Tansy

I stroke Tansy's head as she cuddles next to me. She has been sick during the week. 'A virus of some sort,' the vet said, with a concerned look. The thought of losing my cat sends me into a panic. I have been feeding her chicken broth, and it is working. At last she is breathing normally, the rasping sound gone.

'You'll be fine, my precious,' I whisper to her, and smile as I keep stroking her.

Every pet owner thinks their pet is special, and I'm no different. I am certain that Tansy is exceptionally affectionate and smart with a high "CAT Q". Or at least I think she's extra smart for a cat, and I haven't even mentioned how beautiful she is, with her deep, blue eyes, long, elegant body, two toned coat with seal brown points, and warm, creamy, fawn body.

Recently, I learned some valuable tips from Tansy. I know it seems strange saying that I've learned a lot from a cat. But, as I watched her while she was ill, and then as she recovered, it was a perfect opportunity to do just that. I've been nervous in company since childhood, worried about what others think of me, not wanting to "rock the boat", or thinking of past failures. I was missing out on a lot, not going to parties, scared to try different things or meet new people. But now like many others, I'm constantly searching for new ways to be happier, be well liked and try to do more each day.

A few weeks ago, a job I badly wanted was advertised online, but my fear of not doing well at the interview stopped me from applying for it. I allowed my chance at getting my own claws into work important to me, slip away. If only I had put my nervousness aside, and pushed for what I wanted. Cats have a confidence and purpose that pervades every move they make. Each act is intended. When Tansy wants something, a piece of the chicken I'm cooking, or fish in the fridge, her pupils dilate, and her stare moves between me and the object of her desire. Her focus doesn't shift one bit as she waits to get what she wants. My loud "no" might bring about a temporary shift, but she'll keep trying.

Gradually I will have to take a few more risks, or my life will be dreadfully boring. Cats take calculated risks all the time, jump to high places, leap across distances, enjoying their athleticism. They look effortless and natural as they jump, but they do check height, distance and a place to land before taking the leap.

Perhaps the most important lesson I learned from my cat, is about living in the present. Whether it is enjoying her food or a tummy tickle, she relishes it, and nothing else matters right then. Unlike humans, the last tin of food she ate, and ones in the future are of no concern to her. Of course like all animals, she will remember where the food is kept because knowing that is important. She'll delight in a patch of summer sunlight, or in winter months she'll lie as close as possible to a heater, following what pleases her at that moment. Much of my life is interrupted by a myriad of environmental distractions, chores and a multitude of information to absorb. It would be much more pleasant to relish each moment, be aware of sounds around me, my thoughts and feelings, instead of living in a chaotic rush.

The room is quiet now apart from Tansy's soft purr. I feel her silky fur and some of her bristles as I stroke her coat, and move on to tickle her tummy, listening all the while as her purr deepens. She snuggles closer, at peace… and I am at peace too.

The Seasons

The days become longer and warmer, sudden showers pelt down, as pink and white translucent blossoms dress carpet sidewalks. Bright daffodils, crocuses and tulips show their faces. Fresh, green shoots tell everyone that the delightful season of change, Spring, has arrived, a season to relish in all that is fresh and new. People take long walks, sports begin again, swimmers frolic like ducklings at their first sight of water, and on fields everywhere children are playing.

I have been offered a six week, well-paid, casual job in the city, which puts an end to the walks and picnics I planned. My choice denies me Spring's wonders apart from glances from a car window. I drive along clogged motorways, work through lunch, and return home when it is dark. My attention is concentrated on letters, figures and money. Over the weekend, there are chores to do, and hardly any time for the outdoors.

I am determined to enjoy my day. I rise early to welcome the rosy dawn, as the sun heralds the day. At work, I master the new computer system, take pleasure in brief chats with other workers, enjoy quick cups of coffee and my homemade lunch. During the busy day, I take a few mini breaks, stop to take deep breaths to allow my thoughts to drift to my garden with its falling blossoms. I notice the sounds of chatter, footsteps, and the click of machines. Then I attend to my own sensations of breathing and comfort in my firm chair. No one notices my brief relaxation. Refreshed, I go to the sealed window, look down at the busy city, its lights and people rushing. At the end of my work day, dusk paints the sky in pinks and lavender.

My part-time work is over. Summer awaits. I rise early. It is cool enough for a walk. I am aware of the breeze and feel a quick ripple on my skin. The trees sway exuding a whiff of eucalyptus. The sweet camellias and gardenias in the rich, chocolate soil are flowering, the roses blooming. I stop to inhale their perfumes and admire them.

Back home, I wash dishes, being aware of the water on my hands and the soap bubbles. I listen to the sounds of water running, the squeak of clean plates and jangle of utensils. I do not worry about the past, or what might happen in the future.

My day is full, with work at home, shopping and then meeting a friend. There is just enough time before making dinner for ten minutes of meditation. I turn off the phones and television and sit quietly. With my eyes closed, I drift to my special place, the sea and beach. I walk over warm sand, feel the breeze against my skin again, and watch the waves break.

In the evening, I join my partner for dinner on the patio. We talk, enjoy our food and take pleasure in each other's company as the dark closes around us.

A Positive Way of Life

After searching for a parking spot for ages, at last I find one. With one hand I find my handbag, and with the other I flick my hair into place. I am late again! As I race to the coffee shop to meet my friend Grace, I feel in my bag for my phone, purse and wallet.

We are friends from school days and often meet for coffee. Grace looks attractive, calm and happy, a change from the tense worried woman I had seen just a month earlier.

When I comment on the change in her, and how lovely she looks, she says, 'I've been threatening to do this for ages, but at last I joined a Mindfulness group. I've only been to a few sessions so far, but it's made all the difference. I'm much calmer.'

'Tell me about it,' I ask.

It sounds like another new fad. If it isn't vitamins, it's a magical diet or exercise.

'Mindfulness is a way of feeling more positive about life by being aware of the moment, not living in the past or the future.'

'Mmmmm, interesting!'

At least this sounds helpful.

Grace asks, 'Have you ever been in the car...arrived at your destination, but been unaware of how you got there? Or eaten a chocolate and found it had disappeared without tasting it.'

'It happens to me all the time. I don't understand it.'

'It's like being on autopilot...not being aware of what's happening at the moment in our thoughts, feelings, and other sensations like smell or touch.'

While listening to what Grace has to say about her new fad, I retrieve my phone from my bag. I can't resist checking for messages.

Grace glares at me. 'Trish! The phone has taken over our lives. We're so focused on it that we aren't aware of what's happening around us…and we're missing so much.'

'You're right,' I say. 'I'll turn it off.'

'You haven't been listening.' She sighs.

A habit lately. I wasn't concentrating fully on what she was saying and often don't hear what people are saying.

'Living in the moment…mindfully is important. I have days when I feel down…and you know how much I can worry. Well, Mindfulness has helped me to let all the worry and negatives into my thoughts, accept them for what they are and stop trying to force them out.

'That sounds great. I wish I could do that.'

'I'm still learning, and working on it every day, even doing some meditation.'

I laugh. 'You doing meditation! You swore you'd never ever do it!'

Grace laughs too. 'That was a long time ago. It's actually helping me to feel calmer. I'm trying to do twenty minutes of meditation a day.'

I don't fancy meditation.

'It's the mindful technique that's really helping me,' Grace says.

'Please explain exactly how you do…this Mindfulness…and I won't interrupt again,' I say.

'Especially on down days, and I still have some, I try to be aware of everything I do. When I wake up in the morning, I'm aware of the light in the room, how I feel, the warmth of my body in the bed. I might feel a bit flat or start worrying about things I have to do that day, but I let the thoughts go. When, more positive thoughts start coming, I notice them.

I feel the cool of the tiled bathroom floor, and then the contrast of the soft carpet as I walk to the kitchen. In the kitchen, my phone and television are switched off. I'm aware of smells, sounds, feelings and tastes, as I slowly eat breakfast and savour each mouthful. On bad days when I don't have much of an appetite, I eat what gives me pleasure, whether it's cereal with milk or some fruit.

'I understand what you're saying. I know that I eat fast while thinking of other things, or planning my day. I'm not enjoying my meal…don't even taste it.'

'When I go for a walk later, I'm mindful of the weather, the tress, birds and insects, and the sounds around me. It's been very windy lately and I dislike the wind, but I'm learning that if I'm warmly dressed it doesn't matter much. The wind is doing its work for nature and won't harm me,' she says.

'You're onto something good here Grace. It seems to be helping you.'

'It isn't a fad. I know I've tried lots of different things before, but this works because it's authentic…and it somehow breaks the cycle I get caught up in with multitasking, the phone, Facebook and rushing through the day.'

'Don't I know it!' I laugh.

'You can try it if you like,' Grace says. 'Join my class. Mindfulness isn't magic. It doesn't make worries and down days disappear, but helps to keep me in the present…to live in the "now", and not rake over past stuff, or worry about what could happen in the future.'

'It sounds like a natural, positive way of life. Just what I need.'

Embracing Change

Sea Nymphs

Petros waved to the mystical Sea Nymphs as the ship eased its way out of the harbour. Greeting the Nymphs was a ritual he followed whenever he entered or left a city harbour.

The first time he'd heard about the Nymphs was when he was a child, and his family was emigrating from Greece to Australia, the place they called "The Golden Land". The ship's captain entertained the children on board with Greek legends about these mystical creatures. According to the captain, goddesses of the sea blessed the entrance of the harbour and all crafts that passed through it. He thought nothing of transferring the ancient Greek legends of Poseidon's Nymphs from the Aegean Sea across to the Pacific Ocean. When he produced a worn picture of a Nymph with wispy auburn hair dressed in a white, flowing robe, six-year-old Petros was entranced. His fascination with the mysterious Sea Nymphs continued as an adult whenever he was on the ocean.

As the ship gathered speed, the Sydney harbour became a dot in the background. Petros was on the move again. This time, he was on his way to Hobart. He had visited towns and cities throughout Australia, and further afield. At eighteen when his father died, and six months later his mother died of grief, he left his home in Sydney.

The endless ocean view relaxed him, and filled him with nostalgia. He lit a cigarette, and thought of the house near the beach where he and his family had lived. How he missed them all. After school in almost all types of weather, he and his brothers met up with their school friends on the beach. They competed with each other, racing on the sand, or pitting themselves against giant waves on their surfboards. In the evenings, while his brothers were watching television or "hanging out", he was expected to practice the violin. His parents hoped he would become a violin virtuoso, and insisted on him playing only classical music. Though he delighted in the precision and sound of his instrument, he found the pieces lengthy and difficult. At school, his music teacher had great hopes for his future and clapped loudly whenever he played.

On evenings when his father came home late and his mother was busy in the kitchen downstairs, Petros slipped away to join his friends. Without sufficient practice his playing deteriorated, and when he applied to join the city symphony orchestra he was not good enough. Perhaps if he had been accepted, he may have stayed in Sydney and not taken up an unsettled life of playing popular music in restaurants, or more recently busking on street corners.

On the ship that night, the waters churned and the sky turned mean. In the dark of his cabin, Petros sensed an indefinable presence. He called out, but heard only the sea's roar. A few glasses of red wine helped to still his gnawing uncertainty. When patches of memory plagued him, and familiar voices without names and strains of music wafted past, he finished the first bottle of wine and opened another. Then the Sea Nymphs appeared. Red haired and angry, the plumpest one, seeking attention, spun herself around him so tightly that his chest ached. Another shoved him out of his bunk, insisting he follow her. Reluctantly he obeyed and they drifted together until they reached a bridge deep within a valley. In the undergrowth below lay the twisted wreckage of a car. Instantly he recognised the scene of his father's death. The vile smell of burnt flesh and petrol returned to him. Police swarmed. Passersby gathered. His father's scorched body lay on the grass partially covered by a blanket. Shocked and paralysed with horror, Petros saw himself standing next to the body.

He woke with a headache, but regardless of his drinking the night before, he was certain he had seen the Nymphs. They and other mystical creatures had visited him before. This time he had found them unpleasant, but he conceded that at least they forced him to remember his father's accident and his mother's eyes, red from crying.

The nymphs had delivered an important message. He had avoided thinking about his father's terrible death for far too long. He had not acknowledged how much he missed his parents. And he had not visited their graves. The idea of them lying side by side under the ground marked only by a stone, made him shudder.

Shielding his aching eyes from the bright morning light, he looked out at the calm sea. In about an hour the ship would dock in Hobart. He had visited the small city steeped in nineteenth century colonial architecture, surrounded by a magnificent wild landscape before.

Right then, he felt too unsettled to make a permanent home anywhere. His need to be constantly on the move had insulated him from disturbing thoughts, and even from forming friendships. Women found him attractive, but apart from casual affairs, he discouraged permanency in his relationships. Though many may have envied his interesting and varied lifestyle, his inability to settle, and his fear of attachments did not bring him happiness or peace.

In Hobart Petros managed to find shared lodgings. Then he changed into black striped trousers and a bright red jacket. Once the brim of his hat was set at a jaunty angle he looked every bit the wandering minstrel. With his violin case under his arm, he made his way to an art gallery popular with tourists. He found a spot and entertained one group after another with his repertoire of popular music, light classics and gypsy pieces. His spirited and skilled performance drew the crowds. Every bit the showman, his popularity brought in more money than he expected, but strangely he felt unsatisfied. Though he enjoyed busking, he had to admit to himself that he was drifting through his life without using his true talent and ability. 'Surely I can do better,' he admonished himself.

Once the tourists had left and cruel winter winds stripped the trees, Petros decided to return to Sydney. He gathered his few possessions and his violin, and boarded a ship once more.

As the ship edged out of the harbour he waved to the Nymphs, wondering if they would have another message for him during his journey. He slept restlessly that night and when the Nymphs appeared in a dream, their stay was brief. They kept their distance, except for the large red haired Nymph who pointed her finger at him and waggled it. Then she left hurriedly with the others.

He woke at dawn remembering the Nymph's visit. I think they were telling me that they've done all they can to help me, he mused sleepily. Loud voices and the tempting smell of coffee interrupted his thoughts. He joined the others to brave a wild sea and the spray on deck.

When the ship slowed as the harbour became visible in the distance, he saluted the Sea Nymphs and he whispered, it's about time I made some changes in my life. He rubbed his cold hands together and made two promises to himself. He would practise classical violin daily until he was accepted in a city orchestra, and he would visit his parent's graves. It was time to stop running away. The sun spread it warmth, and he sighed with relief. He felt calmer than he had for long time.

Trapped

Sharon shivered as she looked beyond the bars of her cell onto a bleak, icy day. The concrete of the yard was covered in soupy sleet, and the exercise deprived prisoners were unable to go outside.

Sharon was nineteen, serving two years in prison. Her boyfriend had robbed a bank, and she had driven the "get away" car. With a year served, she faced one more Christmas inside. Though no one had been threatened or hurt in the robbery, and most of the money was returned, she was ashamed that she had been influenced by her boyfriend's greed. She did not blame him for her role in the robbery. Nothing like that would happen again, under any circumstances, she told herself. She didn't read his letters and made up her mind to have nothing further to do with him.

Every day after work in the prison laundry, she paced the yard trying to come to terms with her anger at herself and her guilt. To make matters worse, her mother and sister abandoned her and had not visited her in jail. Her grandmother was the only family member who wrote to her regularly, but she was too ill to visit the jail. Being tossed aside by the rest of her family was her worst punishment.

Initially, Sharon coped with prison life. She was a good listener and had a sense of humour, which made her popular with the guards and her fellow prisoners. But, the confined space, endless routine and severe discipline eventually wore away her resilience. At twilight, the death of the day, work was over. There was nothing to look forward to other than another sleepless night.

One afternoon, the prisoners watched as gardeners cut deep holes in the concrete yard, and filled them with rich earth. They then planted a dozen mature cherry trees. One of the trees stood outside Sharon's cell. There were whispers that the prison governor hoped that the trees would brighten the dull concrete slabs and the mood of the prisoners. The prisoners laughed and joked about the trees. Some even took bets that the trees would bloom before summer, while others bet that they would die before then.

Watching the cherry tree outside her cell grow, brought colour to Sharon's life and helped her to forget her troubles for a while. She talked to the tree often, aware it couldn't hear her and that it had no answers. It was her way of expressing her pent-up feelings. Aware of the tree's every mood in all climates and seasons, she waited for its bare winter skeleton to change. To herald spring, a shower of downy, pink blossoms appeared, and birds and butterflies were attracted to its blossoms. When the tree bore its first cherries, it was almost like the tree's first child. The fruit turned out to be as sweet as she expected.

Gradually she began to view the tree as a prisoner, trapped as she was in the concrete of the yard. She thought that at least when it grew larger, its blossoms would be seen and enjoyed beyond the prison walls.

While the other women spun webs of fantasy and dreams about their future freedom, Sharon was apprehensive about returning to the outside world. On the day of her release, she stood under the cherry tree for a moment, patted its trunk, and then walked through the iron gates of the prison without looking back. The world outside the prison was new and strange, with its busy shopping malls, colours, shapes and smells she had forgotten.

When she visited her grandmother she found her ill and barely coping alone in her home. She was in urgent need of medical attention and practical help. After much discussion, her grandmother decided to sell her house and move into a care facility. Sharon made an extensive search, and found a place for her in an excellent aged home. With all the attention she received and good food, the old lady put on weight, made a few new friends, and seemed far happier. Sharon found part-time work as a cleaner, and was able to spend time with her grandmother.

Sharon's grandmother died three years later, and left her a surprisingly large amount of money. With her inheritance, she bought a plot of land and built a simple house. As soon as she moved into her new house, she bought a large cherry tree similar to the one in the prison yard, and planted it outside her bedroom window. Life without a cherry tree was unimaginable.

Apart from work and shopping, she had no inclination to become involved with the world around her. She was content at home. One crisp spring day when the cherry tree was in full bloom, Sharon received an invitation from her school friend, Marina to visit her farm. The invitation was tempting. After much thought, she decided to go.

She set out for the farm before sunrise. At first she drove hesitantly, unused to being a distance from home. Then she relaxed, enjoying the pastel landscape in the early light. With fresh eyes, she viewed the grasses and trees stirring in the breeze and breathed the sweet morning air. At the farm, the two old friends ate, drank and shared memories. She was given a tour of the farm, the well fed cattle and rows of crops. Marina and her husband were enjoying life, and their farm was a successful venture.

After Sharon's visit to the farm, she realised that it was time for her to edge out of her self-imposed jail. She introduced herself to her neighbours, visited the park and explored further. Gradually she made a few friends. Her memories of jail softened, and she began to enjoy her life.

Once her remaining inheritance was carefully invested, she could live comfortably. During the next three years, she worked as a volunteer at a women's halfway house for ex-prisoners. After long spells in prison the women needed help in adapting to life outside. Through her own experience she assisted many with their day to day problems and finding jobs. But caring and personal experience wasn't enough if she was to help them with their personal and family issues. She realised that she needed to study further, and enrolled in a social work course.

The cherry tree continued to bloom, but Sharon's attitude towards the tree changed. She admired the tree in all seasons and thought of it as an exquisite ornament in her garden.

Three Stones

As Nandi walked along the hilly path to her village the sun hung low in the orange African sky. Sunset was the time of day she liked best, large shadows of trees and bushes accompanying her as evening sounds came alive.

The sharp wintery air made her hungry. Her step quickened as she wondered what her mother would be cooking for dinner. A burst of wind stopped her. She sniffed the air, and shook her head worriedly. Smoke! It wasn't the sweet smoke of food cooking on an open fire. She climbed up onto a rock and looked down on the village. Shocked, she saw huts on the foothills of the mountain burning, including her family's hut. Another group of huts further away were still untouched by fire. Sobbing all the way, she raced home. As she neared the fire, a wall of choking smoke overwhelmed her. With smarting eyes, she searched frantically for her parents, her older sister, and two younger brothers. Everywhere there were charred ruins and the sounds of wailing and weeping. When she reached the blackened, burning embers of what was once her family hut, her uncle held her back forcing her away from the sight of her relatives inside. Both her parents and her sister were dead, but her brothers Sanele aged four and Lwazi eleven, who were playing outdoors when the fire started, were alive and being cared for by members of the tribe. Aunts and cousins stroked Nandi's head, whispered kind words, and tried to comfort her.

The quick action of the men, using simple hoses and buckets to draw water from the river nearby doused the flames and saved some of the huts. Many people had serious burns and were taken to the hospital in the nearest town. Fortunately, the huts of Nandi's uncles and some of her cousins were untouched by the fire.

The terrible task of collecting the fifteen dead tribe members, naming them, and placing them in the coolest spot under the trees, was undertaken by the tribal elders. Only once the dead were buried, the damage could be assessed. Then the reason for the fire was discussed. It was decided that dry grass had caught alight during the evening's cooking, and spread rapidly. No particular person was named or considered to be at fault.

After the ordeal of the burial, Nandi lay limp and exhausted in her uncle's hut, while her brothers sat at her side, waiting for a word or a touch. They were too young to grasp that their parents and older sister would never return. The many sounds around Nandi did not stir her, but eventually the weeping of her brothers roused her. She rose slowly and ate. Gradually she returned to school, and did the schoolwork expected of her in an automatic way. She cleaned the hut and cooked to show her aunt and uncle her gratitude for caring for them all. She neither laughed nor smiled.

At sunset every day, she visited her family's graves. She sat next to the graves, praying for her family's souls until the first star was visible. One evening, the eldest member of the tribe approached her. 'Six months have passed since your loved ones have become part of the earth. It is time for you to go on with your life,' the elder said gently. 'You are fourteen and have a woman's body. Soon you will be ready for marriage and the bearing of many children. Life is to be enjoyed and continued.'

Nandi turned her head away in hurt, but respectfully did not reply. The elder did not understand that the young men of the tribe held no interest for her, and that she could not remember when she had last felt pleasure. The old woman patted her arm and walked away.

Each night, after her evening meal, Nandi joined the other mourners in prayer, but refused to attend tribal gatherings, and stayed in the hut during festivals. She fulfilled the role expected of her by collecting her share of plants and roots, but remained

145

apart from the other women. Instead of spending her free time chatting to friends or playing games, she told her young brothers about their parents and grandparents, and taught them the history of the tribe.

A year later, the old woman found Nandi praying at her family's graves once more. She handed Nandi a finely decorated leather pouch. 'This is a gift from the women of the tribe to help you,' the old woman said kindly.

When Nandi opened the pouch, inside were three coloured stones of different sizes.

The old woman drew her blanket closer against the sharp wind, before pointing to the largest grey stone. 'This stone is for your father, a kind, but serious and powerful man.'

Nandi held the stone to her chest, kissed it and then put it back into the pouch.

The middle round stone had a rusty tone and was smaller than the first one. 'This stone is for your mother who was strong, clever and beautiful.'

Nandi kissed the stone, crying as she held it to her chest before replacing it in the pouch.

The last stone was smaller and pearly white. 'This is for your beautiful, loving sister gone far too young.'

Nandi sobbed as she kissed the stone and held it for a long time before placing it with the others.

'Now your pain is like a knife in your heart, but the hurt will become less as time passes. Keep the stones in the pouch to remember your family until the day comes when you are able to throw them into the river and let them go. Once the pouch is empty, it will always be there for you, as it holds the spirits of your loved ones.'

Nandi nodded her thanks, but did not speak.

After the old woman had left, Nandi sat near the graves long into the night. Several times she opened the pouch, kissed the three stones, and closed it again. Finally, she tied the pouch around her waist. She felt as if her parents and sister were with her again. When she returned to her uncle's hut, she said nothing about the old woman or the pouch, and joined the others near the fire. That night, and for many nights afterwards, she stroked the pouch before she went to bed and slept peacefully.

The winter was long and snow formed on the tall peaks of the mountains. Wild fruits did not grow in the winter, but with the edible roots she had collected and the food her uncle provided, she had sufficient for the boys and herself. At night, she kept her brothers warm in her bed. They were all she had left of her family, and she was determined that they would grow up to be strong, healthy men. She made certain that Sanele went to school each day and she helped her brother Lwazi with his studies, as her mother had helped her.

When the harsh winter had passed, flowers and bright green leaves announced spring. Nandi felt lighter and a little happier. Gradually, she began to chat with her friends and join in with others during tribal festivals. Occasionally, she hummed her favourite songs.

Another year had passed since the death of her parents and sister, and she now visited their graves every second or third day. She remembered the old woman's words. The time had come for her to throw the stones into the river.

At sunset, she went down to the river flowing with spring rains and melted snow. She held each of the stones, turning and kissing them in turn, as she wiped away her tears. When the sky turned navy with its jewel box of stars glimmering, she threw them into the river one at a time. Once the stones had disappeared she prayed that they would find a place of rest. Then she tied the empty pouch around her waist again and walked towards the lights of the tribe. She knew that the day would come when she would remove the pouch to keep amongst her few precious possessions.

The next morning, Nandi woke at peace, knowing that the spirits of her parents and sister would always be with her. She had fulfilled her duty to her brothers, as they were growing up to be strong and happy young men. She went about her chores faster and chatted to her friends. It was time for her to smile and laugh again.

The Winding River

Su Fang's dark eyes brimmed with tears of relief as she surveyed the wide expanse of water. At last she was aboard the sampan. Her search for a new life had begun. In the icy wind, she pulled her woollen cap down over her long, black hair and found a sheltered position. As the craft rocked gently, her thoughts drifted to the events that had led to her journey.

By the time Su Fang was fifteen, her mother had died, her sister had left home to marry, and her two brothers were living in the city. She and her father lived alone in their small house. Their lives followed a predictable routine. Each night they ate a simple meal together. On weekends they went fishing. Each month on a Saturday, they sailed their sampan to the town to buy their few supplies. In their time spent together Su Fang's father often encouraged his daughter's hopes and dreams for the future by saying, 'You are quick, courageous and clever for your age. One day you'll move away from this village and make a good life.' She would smile and nod, but she found difficulty in accepting her father's image of her, or his hopes for her future.

One morning, her father went for his usual walk along the river's edge. Their lives changed when he slipped on the muddy bank, and broke his hip. He was recovering well in hospital, when pneumonia struck. Within a week he was dead. Su Fang mourned for her father and did not leave the house for a month. When she looked in the box where he had kept his money, she found very little. The old sampan was all he had left her of any worth. With no experience to fit her for work, she knew that soon she would be unable to pay the rent on the small house or afford food. Her father had not spoken to his brother for many years, and had told her that he was a mean-spirited man. But, Su Fang had no alternative other than to accept her uncle's offer of food and shelter. Within a week of living with her uncle, her father turned out to be correct. Her uncle treated her like a servant and showed her no respect. She felt alone and trapped in his home, and all her hopes for her future withered.

Each day after completing her chores, she walked along the riverbank. As she grieved for her father, her tears mingled with the water. According to her father's wishes his ashes were scattered on the river, but his spirit visited her several times. She hoped that soon his spirit would find peace and would descend to rest eternally on the river bed.

During a recent visit, his message to her was clear. 'My daughter, leave my brother's home now. Take the sampan and journey along the river to your cousin Wang Hua in the city.'

At first Su Fang ignored the message. Sapped of energy from the day's work and no longer filled with her former zest, she felt unable to fulfill her father's difficult request. But, when her uncle waved a stick in the air threatening to beat her if she didn't work faster and harder, she decided to take her father's advice and leave for the city.

She waited for the Spring, and one morning when pearly light slipped from behind the night clouds, she loaded the sampan with provisions she stole from her uncle's pantry. Then she waded into the icy water. Using all her strength, she pushed the craft into the river.

Su Fang was not afraid of sailing alone. She had lived near the river for many years, and was accustomed to its faces and moods. On the busy river, crafts of all sizes sailed past her. Their owners called greetings and waved. The friendly sailing code of helping each other made her feel secure.

For many days the skies were cloudless with enough of a breeze to sail the sampan along the river. Her journey along the busy river connecting villages to the city was uneventful. At night, her thoughts were of her father and her hope that she would not disappoint him. She recalled often how he had taught her to sail, swim, catch fish, gut them and cook them on a fire.

Su Fang had completed more than half her journey, when the sky darkened, winds swirled and currents raged. The suddenness and ferocity of the storm frightened her. She feared that the small craft would not withstand the storm. Hurriedly, she used the long sculling oar to steer the boat to the river bank. Steering the sampan against the wind in the wild sea was demanding work, but skillfully she managed to secure the boat. Exhausted but relieved, she waited for the storm to pass. Would she manage to reach the city she wondered, as she stared up at the starless sky.

By morning, the storm had almost passed. She was small but strong, and rather than wait for calm, she pushed the sampan back into the water. Several days of pleasant sailing followed until loud banging alerted her. She followed the noise to loose planks. Fortunately, she had her father's metal box that contained basic essentials - a torch, extra batteries, nails, a hammer and twine. Her father had taught her how to mend the sampan. She joined the planks with twine and used nails and the hammer to secure them, hoping that the old sampan would carry her to her destination.

As Su Fang neared the city, she noticed a sampan in the water nearby rocking wildly, and sailed towards it. Two men grappling with a rope called out frantically for help. One of their friends had reeled in what appeared to be a huge fish, when he lost his footing, became entangled in his fishing line, and disappeared into the depths. There was no time for Su Fang to be afraid. Every second counted for the trapped man. She threw off her coat and shoes, and dived into the dark water. What she saw weighing down the line was a long, muscular dragon-fish writhing and kicking to free itself from a fishing hook. Years of fishing had made Su

Fang adept with a rope and knife. Quickly she calculated the best position to make her move. Circling the creature, she distracted it by flicking her shiny knife in front of its eyes. As it ceased its thrashing for a moment, she swiftly threw a rope around it, and pulled tight to immobilise it. Then she cut the snared line to free the relieved fisherman. Together they released the rest of the line, removed the hook and set the dragon-fish free. Pale and exhausted from his terrifying experience, the fisherman thanked Su Fang and applauded her courage.

'Dragonfish… live deep, deep down…and can kill a man,' one of the other fishermen said haltingly.

In recognition for her fast action and courage, Su Fang completed her journey with many sampans sailing alongside as a guard of honour. The extra ripples all the boats created sped her onwards. When at last she saw tall buildings in the distance, she knew that she was nearing her destination.

Finding her cousin Wang Hua in the city involved asking many people and a great deal of searching, but at last they were united. They had been close as children, and were delighted to be together. Wang Hua's family welcomed Su Fang, and she now had a new home.

In the weeks and months that followed, Su Fang noticed a change in herself. Though her courage was known to all those on the river and some further afield, it was her view of herself that had changed. Her journey had shown her that she knew that she could do most things if she applied herself. Her experience as her uncle's unskilled servant had also made her realise her need to study further.

Now that his daughter no longer needed his guidance, the spirit of Su Fang's father sank to the riverbed where he rested forever. The dragon-like creature was never seen on the river again.

Across the Bridge

The old man hobbled through the windy alley towards the bridge. He passed awnings, dark corners he had shared with stray cats, and garages where he had spent many nights. When his wife died two years earlier, he lost himself, and now nothing mattered other than joining her. His children cared about him and had begged him to live with them, but in his grief, he had refused. Later, when they searched for him they could not find him.

At the bridge, he struggled up the steps. 'Things will never change,' he muttered with an exhausted sigh, as he held onto the rails unsteadily. His frail body slid down to the wooden boards, and he lay there not bothering to find a more comfortable position. Shimmering lights across the river beckoned, but he was unaware of them, or the moored fishing boats bobbing in the distance. He saw only the swirling, welcoming water below. After fumbling, he found his flask. With one slug he emptied it. 'Soon I'll be with her and at peace.'

The lapping water lured him into sleep. When he awoke to a sky of gilt and rose, he muttered angrily to himself. He had already missed his opportunity to escape his misery. The early risers were crossing the bridge. Some passers-by laughed and pointed at him. Others pitied him and threw coins in his direction, but he was unaware of them all. He battled to stand, hoping to move to a more secluded spot, but too weak, he sank in defeat.

Sleep overcame him again, until children on their way home from school rushed past his huddled figure. He cursed their pounding feet and noisiness. Noticing the wintry blast for the first time, he shivered, buttoned his coat, and wrapped his scarf around his chest. When squeaks and movement across his body alerted him, he pulled himself into a sitting position. 'Filthy rats!' he sneered. With a fast flick of his hand across his matted coat, they scurried off.

In the mellow, afternoon light, he noticed flocks of birds darkening the sky. Further along the bridge, a boy and his father were fishing. He watched them. And after almost an hour they had caught nothing, until with a yell of delight the boy tugged at his line. He had hooked a large wriggling fish. Though the father urged his son to throw the fish back into the water, the boy shook his head.

With the fish in his hand, the boy ran up to the old man. 'For you,' the boy said shyly as he offered his catch.

Suddenly hungry, the old man grabbed the fish. 'Thanks,' he said in a rough whisper, as he wiped away his tears of gratitude. He sucked the fish's moisture and ate the raw flesh. He then closed his eyes in contemplation. The boy reminded him of his son at the same age.

As the sky turned vermillion, he was aware of the people crossing the bridge on their way to the city's many theatres, bistros and cafes. There were kind looks and nods in his direction, with the occasional word of encouragement, as well as a few mean remarks.

The rush of water below was no longer enticing. After looking up at the evening star and pale moon, gingerly he tried to stand. With a few attempts, he found his balance. Holding onto the rail tightly he shuffled across the bridge towards the lights across the river, where his children lived.

The Blue Venetian Jar

Nina had finished work for the day. She applied lipstick, fixed her hair, and though it was warm, she put on her coat to cover her body. She had gained a little weight and felt self-conscious. Before catching her bus home, she wandered into the shopping mall. As a heat surge overwhelmed her, creating two pink patches on her cheeks, she peeled off her coat. As she soaked up beads of perspiration, she sighed, resenting the changes in her body. Her youth was gone, she thought, and she felt less of a woman.

A shop tucked into a corner of the mall caught her attention. A few pieces of pottery and some bric-a-brac were attractively arranged in the cramped window. She stepped inside to view the once-loved treasures more closely, an ornate silver brush and comb set, a tapestry footstool, fancy cups, plates and familiar ornaments that stirred her memory of days past and people now gone. A white fluted dish with a braided handle caught her eye, and she smiled. Her great aunt Davina once owned a dish just like it and kept it filled with sweets and chocolates. A group of tiny figurines reminded her of her grandmother's prized collection of miniature ornaments kept behind glass in a prominently placed dresser in the sitting room. As a child, she was fascinated by a tiny pair of blue and gold shoes and a dancing lady that fitted into the palm of her hand.

While admiring a blue vase, she experienced another prickly wave of heat. In her haste to cool herself by pulling up the sleeves of her jumper, she knocked over the vase. It lay shattered on the floor. Though she rarely cried, tears trickled down her cheeks. The unusual intensity of emotion and the uncomfortable changes she was undergoing, had begun a few weeks earlier.

As the shop owner swept up the glass, Nina's tears subsided. She calmed herself, stood awkwardly for a while, and then looked around the shop. She decided to buy an old ginger jar. Once she had paid for the jar and the broken vase, she rushed to the bus stop.

That evening, when she unwrapped the jar, she noticed a flaw in the pattern. One stem of leaves pointed in the opposite direction to all the others. She liked the jar and wasn't concerned about its pattern. After moving the jar around the room, she was satisfied that the best place for it was on top of the wooden cabinet in front of a decorative mirror. Curiosity tempted her to lift the jar's lid. Inside was a dried posy of strawflowers and a few forget-me-nots, tied with a faded, red, satin ribbon. Carefully she lifted the posy. It was old, but its faded petals had survived. She turned it about in her hand and wondered who had hidden it there. Perhaps a young woman had received it from an admirer.

As she replaced the lid, she glanced at her reflection in the mirror. She had put on too much weight, her skin was still moist and unwrinkled, but her expression was tense. She disliked the image she saw. 'In time my face will dry and fade like the flowers in the jar.'

During the next few days, she thought about the second jar she had noticed at the shop and that it would make an attractive partner to the first one. At the end of that week, she finished work a little earlier and hurried to the shop. She found the jar she wanted and took it to the counter. The owner of the shop was busy with a customer. While she waited, she watched the shop owner's young daughter playing on the floor with a smiling clown figurine.

'That's a lovely clown,' Nina said to the girl.

The girl nodded. 'He's my favourite… and Mum saved him for me,' the girl said.

'Oh! How did she do that?' Nina said, bending to look at the clown more closely.

The girl looked away remembering. 'Last year, I dropped him on the floor and he broke into lots of tiny pieces. I couldn't stop crying, so Mum stuck all the bits together until he was fixed.'

'You must've been very relieved about that.' Nina smiled.

'Yes...but when the lady who comes to clean the house was dusting, she knocked him off the shelf. I thought he was broken for good this time and couldn't be fixed.' She stroked the figurine. 'But he was so well stuck together that he was extra tough and didn't break.'

'Maybe that's why he's got such a big, happy grin,' Nina said to the girl.

When Nina made her purchase, she asked the owner of the shop about the flaw in the pattern of the jar she had bought earlier.

'Some painters make mistakes on purpose. It's their way of showing that they aren't perfect.'

Nina was disappointed to find that the pattern on the second jar was flawless, and that nothing had been hidden in it. When she placed the pair of jars together on the cabinet, they looked especially attractive.

Weeks later, she had a dream about the shop. It was a hot night and the atmosphere was oppressive. Objects she had seen displayed were in a circle in the moonlight. The sweet dish was bursting with sweets and chocolates, the figures and both jars were there too. The imperfection on the first jar formed a strikingly lovely pattern. The other jar was filled with fresh strawflowers tied with a red, satin ribbon. The child's clown figurine danced and pulled funny faces. Nina was in the dream too, looking confident and happy. A streak of moonlight caught the lovely blue Venetian vase that she had dropped. It was now whole again.

She awoke from the dream feeling rested. It was her first peaceful night without drenching sweats. Perhaps the real change is beginning, she thought. *Becoming older is an important phase in my life. The wrinkles and slight weight gain aren't that important. I have so much to look forward to and I am going to enjoy it.*

157

The Rose Garden

Darren's administrative job was secure and he earned a good salary, but each day he dreaded going to work. The repetitive nature of his work had bored him for the last five years. Though he longed for more challenge and creativity at work, he remained with his safe job as his father had suggested. At almost forty-five, he feared he had left changes in his occupation too late.

During the warmer months, Darren found pleasure and expression for his creativity in his garden. He designed an imaginative retreat that boasted tall trees, flowers, native shrubs, an expanse of lawn, as well as hothouse. In the hothouse he grew orchids and tropical plants.

That Spring, he decided to plant a rose garden at the side of the house. He chose twenty-eight rose bushes that the nursey man said would do well in open sunlight or part shade. As he planted them, one particular rose excited him, an intensely fragrant hybrid tea rose called Valencia. It was long stemmed with large, creamy blooms suffused with apricot. As he sniffed the Valencia he closed his eyes transported with delight. While the other roses were beauties, he decided to place this particular rose in the hothouse where he could give it extra care.

The summer brought a few scorching days followed by several heavy rain storms, unusual for that time of year. Most of the plants in the garden stood up to the challenging weather, including the rose bushes that grew larger and flowered abundantly. Soon he would have a magnificent rose garden. But in the hot house with the constant temperature and moisture, the Valencia rose wasn't growing at the rate of the outdoor plants, and though it flowered its blooms were small.

Darren's asked his neighbor, an experienced gardener, for help. 'Too much water and not enough air in there,' his neighbour said. 'Put the rose outdoors and show it off. It's a pity to lock it away.'

Darren was reluctant to risk putting the Valencia outdoors to face the elements as it was his favourite plant, but after thinking about it, he planted the rose outdoors with the others. After a period of adjustment, the rose flourished and soon flowered with big, billowing blooms.

When his neighbour saw the rose in its prime he commented. 'Only goes to show how important it is to think through things carefully and then take a few risks. The plant might have withered away if you hadn't moved it.'

That night as Darren lay awake, he thought about the rose bush and his job. Perhaps it was time to move on, to take a few calculated risks. He wondered why he had taken his father's advice to stay in his safe job. After all he was nothing like his father. His mother was the creative one, who loved flowers and gardens, and at seventy she was still doing new things. Perhaps like his favourite flower, he was more resilient than he thought. It was time to find out if he could come out into the sunshine.

Overcoming Obstacles

Whale Song

Gina took the long route home from university, along the slopes covered with fallen Autumn leaves and flame tinged trees, towards the curve of the beach. Whenever she was sad or worried the sea and stretch of beach helped to calm her. It was also a place where she met her friends, celebrated, and had fun in the water.

She was a music student at university, who had played the flute from the age of six. She practised daily with the hope of becoming a professional flautist. That morning, she had played her flute in an exam. She was disappointed in her playing, and the beach was the place she went to for solace. Gina's tutors saw a positive future for her. They were impressed by her technical skill and her sensitive interpretation of the music, but they were concerned about her self-consciousness, that interfered with her playing for an audience. She was young and in her first year of study. They were certain she would overcome her difficulties.

While walking on the beach, Gina was so absorbed in scolding herself about her playing, that she almost collided with an elderly man.

He lifted his arm in a mock stop sign. 'Hey, watch it young lady! Where are you rushing to?'

She mumbled a quick apology.

'Slow down! Nothing is worth the rush.'

The concern on his wrinkled face and gentle tone of his voice soothed her. She smiled in thanks, and walked away slowing her pace.

During the cool, windy days of Autumn, warmly dressed children made sandcastles on the beach, surfers and only the bravest swimmers were in the water. Near a group of rocks she noticed a crowd had gathered and were gazing out at sea. She assumed that they were hoping to spot whales. The news had spread that two whales and their calves had been sighted close to the shore line earlier that morning.

In Autumn, whales migrated from the icy Antarctic to warmer Australian waters to give birth to their young. Occasionally they came close to the shore. When the young whales had grown large enough they returned to the Antarctic to mate.

She scrambled up the tallest rock, the best viewing spot, shook the tendrils of her dark hair from her face and waited. Cheers from the crowd below announced their sighting of two whales and their calves. Excitedly she watched the spectacle of one of the whales breaching. The huge mammal raised its tail, its flukes clearly visible, and then made a second and third acrobatic breach. Amazed by its power, size and fluid movement, she throbbed with excitement. She watched the whales play until the sun dipped on the horizon.

The following day, Gina visited the beach again. The water was calm and the sand glowed in the pale sunlight. She strolled towards the rocks again, but no whales were visible. When she found a warm spot with an uninterrupted view of the sea, she delved into her carry bag for her flute. Facing the sea she began to play. The haunting sounds carried across the sand. Lost in playing, she was unaware of the growing number of people drawing closer. When she stopped, she was stunned by the crowd and their appreciative clapping.

I'm not even nervous. If only I can play as well at the recital in a few weeks.

Her audience called out "more, more" and she played a medley of popular tunes. The old man she had almost knocked over was in the front of the crowd, smiling at her.

'You play beautifully…almost like the whales singing,' he said. She was surprised.

'Listen to the song of the whales…they'll delight you.'

Later, Gina searched for videos of "singing" whales on her computer. The old man was correct. She was enthralled by the rich, haunting vibrations. Each whale had its own "song" in a range of octaves, just as each flautist had an individual style of playing. Fascinated, she read articles about the way in which whales communicate. She discovered that they swim alone or in pairs. In order to navigate, detect food or warn each other of danger, they have a special way of connecting with each other over many kilometres.

She was so captivated by whale sounds that when she next visited the shopping mall she bought recordings of whales and dolphins, accompanied by flutes. Over the next few weeks, Gina prepared for the recital at the university. She had been given a solo part, and was both excited and nervous. For relaxation each night, she listened to the whales and dolphins with flutes in the background, and then rehearsed her piece.

If those huge creatures can communicate, and be aware of each other so superbly, I can reach my audience. I will imagine I'm a whale, calling to a mate when I play and forget about myself.

During the recital she was nervous at first, but her nerves left her as she focused on her own playing, as well as the rest of the orchestra. She felt herself reaching out to her audience and at the end of the recital the audience responded with a standing ovation.

Early the following morning at dawn, Gina ran to the beach. At the water's edge she played her flute hoping that the whales could hear her message of thanks.

Inspiration Fired

Erin lived alone in a cottage on the fringe of a town that nestled at the foot of the mountains. As her grandmother had done before her, she tended to a large garden with a variety of flowers and a field of vegetables. Some of the produce she kept, and the rest she sold at the village market. Apart from the pleasure gained in working with the rich earth, admiring the colours of the delicate blooms and sniffing their scents, nothing interested her. She carried the burden of a heavy ache, barely noticing whether the sun shone brightly, or it rained. She raked the ground, turned the soil and planted seedlings automatically. Her parents had been killed by a landslide when she was little, and her elderly grandmother died when she was in her late teens. She was an only child, alone and disconnected from the world. Without the confidence to talk to strangers or seek friendships, her interest lay in a rich fantasy life.

Erin's daydreams of a warm and loving mother began when she started school. She dreamed of a mother who smiled and waved when she went off in the morning, and kissed her when she returned. Then a caring teacher became a focus of her fantasies. When the teacher became pregnant, Erin watched her round tummy growing, and imagined she was inside it, warm and wanted. She missed the teacher when she left to have her baby, but her daydreams about the baby's birth, and even the room it slept in continued to dominate her thinking. She visualised a pastel pink room with candy striped curtains, a white bassinette and a huge, cuddly teddy bear. Later, when Erin grew into a woman, other fantasies of being in a loving environment developed, and she filled her thoughts with an imaginary husband and family based on pictures she had seen in magazines.

One year, fierce rains and swirling winds swamped the flowers and uprooted the vegetables. Erin feared she would starve during the winter. Unused to dealing with such huge practical problems, she did nothing but stare at the sodden ground and sigh. When her store of food was almost eaten, her reaction was to think wildly of escape. She thought of climbing to the highest point of the nearby hill and throwing herself into the ravine below. During restless nights she dreamed of her dead body lying rotting and undiscovered in the ravine.

Hunger woke her early one morning, and she ate the last bit of bread. She paced the small sitting room until that afternoon, when suddenly fired with energy, she hurried to the forest. Patches of bright berries grew under the tall canopy of trees. She picked handfuls and stuffed them into her mouth. Then she looked for roots and leaves that her grandmother had taught her were safe to eat. After she had eaten her fill, she collected fruits, mushrooms, yams and roots to cook and eat later. Before leaving, she sat in a sunny spot and admired the lushness around her.

She woke the following day with a novel idea. 'Perhaps I could put a posy together of all the lovely branches and plants in the forest and sell them at the market.' It seemed like a silly idea, and she pushed it away.

A few days later, she returned to the forest with her basket. After filling her basket with mushrooms and wild yams, she went deeper where tall pines, spruces and beeches grew. Inspired by the beauty of the trees, she collected pine cones, and cut branches to put in her basket.

The yams and mushrooms made a tasty stew and sustained her, as she worked furiously putting the leaves and branches together in posies. Her imagination was stirred, and there was no room for fantasy that night. Trying this way and that, she assembled branches, cones and leaves attractively, and added lace and velvet ribbons from her grandmother's old sewing basket to decorate the posies she had made.

166

Hours later, she woke feeling uncertain. Who will want my posies? I doubt I'll sell any. In spite of her apprehension, she arrived at the market early. Initially there was no interest in what she had to sell, but by mid-morning when the town's ladies came to market, they were fascinated with her unusual creations.

'Aren't they lovely, so different. My posy will go nicely in my living room,' she heard one say.

Another woman told her friend, 'A perfect gift.'

Nearly all her posies were sold and Erin went straight to the store to buy food.

'How creative and imaginative you are,' a woman at the store said. 'I'd never have thought of taking a few leaves and putting them together in that way.'

Erin walked back to the cottage, her mind charged with ideas. I could pick flowers that grow in the forest, tie them up and hang them to dry from the rafters in the kitchen. They will make lovely, delicate arrangements that I could sell too, she thought.

She sold her posies of branches and dried flowers until she had saved sufficient money to restore her ravished garden. She bought rich topsoil, spread it liberally, and scattered seeds over the ground. With rain and sunlight her garden flourished and fresh food was plentiful again. By now, her plant decorations and fresh produce was selling well. She couldn't manage the increased workload alone and employed young people from the village on a casual basis. She was making a good living and enjoying creating innovative decorations from forest flowers, leaves and branches. Though her confidence grew as demand for her products increased, she remained shy, only answering questions her buyers asked. But, in bed at night, she imagined long friendly conversations with the people she met at the market.

Over the months that followed, she gradually became confident enough to talk more freely to people. Later she accepted invitations from neighbours, who were inspired by her ideas. She experimented making new arrangements from the flowers and trees around her, enjoying her newfound creativity.

Erin's inner ache eased at last and her life began to take on a new positive direction.

Midlife

It was 6.05 p.m. in a bar in the city. Anton was perched on the edge of his stool waiting for his uncle Janos, who worked a few blocks away. The two men met regularly for a chat at the bar after work, as they found it easier to talk away from their wives and children. At thirty-eight, Anton was handsome with dark hair, an olive complexion and expressive, brown eyes that reflected his every mood. He was dressed in a dark suit and striped tie that matched his pastel shirt. Janos, seven years older, rushed in with apologies for being late. His grey hair was tousled, his face lined and his clothing was casual.

They ordered a beer and enquired about the health of each other's family.

Anton sighed and stared at the floor.

Janos looked at Anton quizzically. 'What's up with you?' 'I've been feeling down lately and I don't know why,' Anton replied slowly.

'Anything I can do to help?'

Anton rubbed his manicured hands that had not seen manual work for some time. 'It doesn't make sense, but I'm bored managing the company. I would love to get my hands in the soil again. I haven't touched it for years, and I miss it.'

'I was young when we left Cyprus, but I remember the farm back there, the veggie gardens, wheat and goats. I've been back, but it's a modern farm now with lots of technology,' Janos replied. 'At this stage of my life I'm not interested in farms. I've got my eye on a second hand car I've seen. It's an M.G, a beauty!'

The two men sat in silence as they sipped their beers.

Anton commented, 'We've both been fortunate. Our parents saved to give us a good education. I think I've achieved what they wanted, and what I thought I wanted, but now I'm not so sure. I'm restless.'

Anton didn't tell his uncle that he had been drinking more whisky than usual, and that he was smoking weed every night, something he had not done since his student days.

Janos nodded. 'Yeah, our parents sacrificed a lot for us.'

Anton sighed. 'I'm feeling locked into my job in the city now… with no way out.'

Janos smiled ruefully. 'Don't I know it! I'd like to work nearer home and have more time for other things.' He took a gulp of beer. 'If it's a small farm you're after, you could buy a small holding not too far from the city. The kids would love it over weekends, but I'm not so sure about Barbara.'

'We've looked at a few places, and you're right, she's not that keen on a farm, but she wouldn't stop me,' Anton said. Janos placed another round of beer on the table. 'Think about it, Anton, if it's important to you, it counts.'

'Sure.'

After a few moments Anton looked at his uncle. 'I've been having some weird dreams lately…all similar. I don't know what to make of them. Do you have any interesting dreams?'

Janos sipped his drink. 'Na, I sleep like the dead, but come on, share them.'

Anton looked down, a little embarrassed. 'This is the dream I had two nights ago.'

I was under a tree in a barren field, shivering from cold. The sky turned dark and the atmosphere was oppressive. Then suddenly, a gold band spread across the sky. A sound disturbed the branches. I looked up and saw a magnificent bird with a sapphire body and huge wingspan. It flitted and swooped until it settled on a low branch so close to me that I could see it pulsating with energy. I asked myself if the bird had come to lift me up and carry me away.

'Then I woke up.' Anton scratched his head. 'It's a strange dream and I don't have a clue about dreams. Our *Ya Ya* would've known. She was amazing at interpreting dreams.'

Janos struggled to find the right words. 'Maybe you need a break. Take a long holiday and I'm sure you'll feel better.'

Anton took his uncle's advice. He and Barbara went on a Mediterranean cruise. While they were enjoying themselves, Barbara's parents cared for their two children. On the days when the ship was anchored they took sightseeing trips. As their tour bus traveled through the countryside they passed several farms. Anton wished the bus would stop at just one of the farms long enough for him to walk around and smell the earth, see the crops growing and the animals.

Anton returned to work with renewed energy, but it wasn't long before he dreamed about the farm and the bird again. To understand more about his dreams, he bought a dream book, but he found no answers in it and tossed it into a cupboard.

While he was walking his dog late one afternoon, he saw his elderly neighbour, Mrs. Randall, in her garden. She was attempting to prune shrubs, but in the process almost fell over.

He rushed to her aid. 'Are you alright, Mrs. Randall?' She looked exhausted and her arms were scratched.

Tears filled her eyes. 'I'm desperately trying to tidy my garden. My children say that the house with its big garden is too much for me to handle. They're nagging me to sell and move into a retirement village. I can manage the house, but the garden has run wild. I want to prove to them that I'm not senile and can manage it all. I love this place and its memories, and I'd hate to leave. You know, I lived here with my parents as a child. When I married Jack we made it our home and brought our children up here.'

'I remember your husband and children well,' he replied.

'Jack was very fond of you, Anton.' She snapped off the top a dead flower. 'I know I could hire a gardener, but I'm afraid of having strangers on my property. At my age it's not safe.'

'Don't worry Mrs. Randall, I'll get the garden in shape for you. I enjoy gardening. It'll be my pleasure.'

Two weeks later, Janos and Anton met at the bar once more.

'You're looking well and happy. Another one of your dreams? I can tell by your smile,' Janos said, as he opened his bottle of beer.

Anton laughed. 'You know me well.'

'Well, out with it then.' Janos's eyes sparkled with amusement.

This time I was in a forest where flowers, fruit and wild plants of all colours grew. The perfumes and buzz of insects around me was so exhilarating that I lost my way back to the path. I was tired from battling to find my way, and sat on the grass under a tree and rested. I felt so happy and free. It was wonderful!'

'Ah! It was such a lovely dream…short though.' Anton said with a sigh.

'Yeah, it was.' Janos said, as he tried to find a more comfortable position on the small stool. 'Whatever it means it's happier than the last dream you told me about eh!' He smiled, and gave Anton a nudge.

Anton told his uncle that he had been helping Mrs. Randall with her garden. 'It's overgrown and almost wild in parts, but I'm enjoying working with the earth and plants. It's strange that as I worked I could sense a warm presence in the background.'

'You've taken on a big job for that old lady,' Janos said, raising his eyebrows.

'I don't mind at all. Working in her garden has been fun. She's a lovely lady. I don't want her children to push her out of her home.'

Janos moved his glass around on the table before replying. 'Well, it's doing you good, far better therapy than those tablets people take.'

Anton laughed and talked on excitedly. 'I planted some new flowers as a gift for Mrs. Randall. When she saw her garden she was speechless and hugged me.'

'You've done a good deed!' Janos lifted his glass to his nephew.

'You know, as I was tidying the last few grass cuttings on the lawn before leaving, I heard a fluttering sound in the tree nearby and felt a soft breeze. Don't think I'm crazy, but I thought it could've been the bird I dreamed about.'

Janos nodded but didn't comment.

'Even if I imagined the bird, it helped me. I feel more positive about my life, and that the future holds hope for me now.'

'I'm pleased for you,' Janos gave Anton a slap on the shoulder. 'Sometimes things like this happen for a reason. We don't always have to understand them.'

'I've left my good news for last,' Anton said. Barbara is so pleased to see me looking happy again that we've agreed to use the inheritance from my father as a down payment on a small farm. She knows I will enjoy working my own land like my family have over the centuries,' he said with a grin.

Janos slapped the table and drank the last of his beer. 'Just like the old days, eh? I'll turn up to your farm in my new car, but don't ask me to plant anything.'

The Pottery Mug

Robyn's administrative job was secure, she earned a good salary, but she was bored by the repetitive nature of her work. Though she longed for more challenges, she stayed in her safe job. At almost forty-five, and a single mother of two daughters, she thought she had left any occupational changes too late.

The friends she'd made at work eased her dissatisfaction. Benita who worked in the same office became a close friend. Over a sweltering weekend, Robyn, Benita and both their families held a picnic on a river bank. After lunch, Benita's husband took the children fishing. The two women sat chatting in the shade with their legs dangling in the cool water. Benita told Robyn about the art class she was attending. She enjoyed the classes and had surprised herself by producing paintings her family and friends admired.

'I look forward to my classes every week. If I'm bored at work, I spend a few moments thinking about a painting I'm working on. I can't wait to get home to try a new colour or to make a change to it.'

Robyn smiled warmly. 'That's great Benita!, I've noticed that you're looking happy lately.'

'My work doesn't sap my energy or stress me like it did before… there's my art when I'm home. Of course there are chores too, but I've insisted that the children help out more,' she said with a smile, as she threw a twig into the water and watched it drift away.

'I'm being honest, I'm envious. My job frustrates me,' Robyn said with a sigh.

'Join our art group. You never know, you might have artistic talent,' Benita said.

'I can't draw...never could. It would be a waste of time,'

Benita touched her friend's arm gently. 'Well, something else then. There are so many fun things to enjoy outside work.'

A month later on another hot day, the air conditioning at work broke down. Robyn left the office earlier than usual and went straight to the cool shopping mall. She bought an iced drink and wandered past the shops. She stopped to admire a display of handmade pottery. There were bowls, mugs, plates, as well as sculptures of animals and plants. Intrigued, she entered the shop to have a closer look. The decorative fruit bowls would look magnificent on her table, she thought. She lifted up a large one and felt the texture.

While Robyn was trying to decide which piece to buy, another customer was admiring the pottery as well. 'Wonderful work isn't it? I wish my own efforts at pottery were half as good,' the woman said.

'You do pottery too?' Robyn asked.

'I go to a pottery class, but I'm not that good. Enjoyment is the main thing for me.'

'Oh yes! It must be fun.'

The two women discussed making pots, then Robyn said, 'Would you mind me asking where you go for pottery classes?'

'We're a small group but there may be room for one more.' The woman looked in her handbag for a slip of paper and a pen, and wrote down a name and address. 'I hope you'll join us,' she said, handing the note to Robyn.

Robyn thanked the woman and left the shop with a carefully wrapped decorative bowl.

Robyn kept the details about the pottery group in her purse, but didn't phone for more information until weeks later. She had doubts that she would be able to produce anything creative. She thought that she was a practical person who had never made anything unusual or interesting.

On the morning of her birthday, she received phone calls, emails and cards with good wishes, as well as presents from her children. When she arrived at work, a huge wrapped parcel lay on her desk. Excitedly she tore away the paper. It was a beautiful landscape painting signed by Benita. Before she could find her friend to thank her for the gift, people working near her gathered to look at the painting. Everyone wished her "happy birthday" and commented on her luck at receiving such a lovely present.

At home, Robyn placed Benita's painting on the wall above the table where the new pottery bowl stood. Together they enhanced the room.

'Come on, try something creative,' Benita said to Robyn when they met for coffee one afternoon after work. 'What's the worst thing that could happen?'

'I'll be useless, make an idiot of myself.'

'So what!' Benita laughed.

'You're right,' Robyn smiled. 'Nothing terrible would happen.'

Two weeks later, Robyn attended the first of many Saturday classes at the pottery group. Initially, she was nervous and clumsy, but she enjoyed the soft, squishy feel of the clay. She began hand building plates by working the clay into shape. Then she learned how to throw the clay on the pottery wheel. She made mugs and platters, and decorated them. Once they came out of the kiln, she was amazed. The mugs would be useful at home, and they were more attractive than she had imagined. Impulsively she decided to surprise Benita. Her friend was thrilled to find a gift of a mug on her desk.

The best part was that she enjoyed the pottery classes so much that her job no longer frustrated her. When her work bored her, she found time to think about her pottery. She planned to make matching plates, bowls and cups, an entire set. She was able to work out colours and designs when she took short breaks on the computer. She was delighted when her boss commented on how much happier she seemed and that she was quicker and more accurate in her work.

She had solved her problem in a least expected way.

Flowing Freely

Karen put her paintbrush down and gazed critically at her dull canvas. It lacked the vitality and strength of her other paintings. Painting usually lifted her mood, fired her imagination, but this time it wasn't working for her.

I haven't finished a painting for two weeks. This one doesn't look as if it's going to be any good either. With this dry spell, how am I going to have enough work for an exhibition at the end of the year?

She shook her head despondently and left her studio. As she dressed, she glanced at herself in the mirror. *I've put on a lot of weight and I look awful.*

Flattening her stomach with her hand, she rebuked herself for not eating slimming, healthy foods, or exercising as she had promised herself.

In the kitchen she poured a cup of coffee and thought about her predicament.

It's no good staring at the canvas and worrying. I'll take my bike out. I might lose some weight and a fun ride could give me the inspiration I need to help with my painting.

The sky was cloudless, the day warm, as Karen rode out of the suburbs, enjoying the sensation of the wheels spinning beneath her. She peddled energetically through lush greenery and past tall trees, aware of the soothing hum of insects and birdcalls. Occasionally she stopped to admire birds, or plants.

I wish I'd brought a sketch pad and pastels along to capture all the magnificently coloured and interesting details around me.

Tired, she stopped to place her bicycle against a tree. After her rest she walked about admiring the many birds. Almost hidden by a tall clump of trees was a clear, sparkling pool edged with ferns. The water was so inviting that she stripped, untied her braided hair, and waded in. Luxuriating in the cool, she floated like an exotic flower with only the ripples from her slight movements disturbing the water's smooth surface.

When reluctantly she stepped out of the pool, she saw her reflection in the water's mirrored surface. At first, she saw herself as a mischievous young girl slipping back into the water like a seal. She was athletic and sensual then, and young men were attracted to her.

Then, her adult self appeared. She looked at her unsmiling image with her mother's critical eyes and recoiled. Her mother was stick thin, and had expected her to be thin too. Daring to look again, she held her breath as she looked more carefully at the attractive face, shining eyes, and well-proportioned figure shimmering before her. This time she liked what she saw, a full breasted, sensual nude.

I'm rubenesque, like the women Peter Paul Rubens once painted…curvaceous and earthy. That's me, not a doubt. I'm not meant to be skinny. Just thinking of Ruben's superb paintings of sensual nude women makes me happy.

Her long hair dried in the sun, flowing freely, as it cascaded over her naked shoulders. She lay back relishing the warmth on her body, aware of a new optimism surging through her.

When the sun disappeared behind the mountains and the air cooled, she dressed reluctantly and rode home. Along the route she marveled at the long purple shadows and the darkening trees that cast a silhouette against the tangerine sky. Her mind was bursting with images of the sunset, the forest and the leafy pool.

I will create something magnificent when I paint all this on canvas and I'll have enough paintings for my exhibition.

Sebastian's Diary

Sebastian is an incredible cat who lives with Shane and Hannah. He writes a diary about a difficult period in his life.

Day One

Purrrrfect! My diary starts today on my birthday. I'm two years old, but no presents for me yet from my Humans. When I was sixteen-weeks-old, I was stolen from my mamma and brought here by my Humans, a "He" and a "She". They call me Sebastian, but I am also their Beautiful, Good Boy, Treasure, Precious, Sweetie and Sweetheart. If they are not pleased with me they call me Naughty Cat. It depends on their mood. There are some Little Ones who visit sometimes, and try to pull my ears and tail, but I hide from them under the bed. I've taught my Humans my ways and most times I get what I want, and extra cuddles too. They have learned quite well.

Now I'm in a sun spot near the window and watching. A little dark thing is creeping across the floor. I can reach it without having to move. Easy does it…my paw strikes out…got it! Bite its head off…but it tastes muuuughh!

I stretch and roll on my back. Time to check my house. In and out I go, rub and leave my mark on corners, doors, and furniture. Roll on the carpet to make sure everything has my scent. I know I must not spray or they will go crazy.

There's one place I won't go…to Jasmine's room. It still has her smell. The house was Jasmine's when I arrived here, and there was no place for me. She turned her head away, flicked her tail, growled and hissed at me. Jasmine ate my food and pissed in my water, but she was beautiful and she knew it. Creamy all over except for her boots, the tips of ears and tail. Her blue eyes were even bluer than the sky on a clear day. She was always the top cat, but she got used to me, even loved me. No more thinking about Jasmine now. I'm missing her too much.

I'm listening to His heavy steps coming to open the curtains to let in the lovely, warm light. Her quick steps follow. 'Where are you my precious,' She calls.

I stretch and stretch again, pretending not to hear.

'Come, my Sweetie.'

I walk to her slowly.

'Happy birthday Sebastian my sweetheart …two-years-old today!' She picks me up and holds me tightly in her arms and kisses the top of my head.

I struggle to get away. I hate being picked up and held. She should know that by now! She lets me go. I shake myself free.

'I have a lovely gift for you,' She says.

It's a stick with a dark, furry thing at the end. Mmmmm! It doesn't look much, but one swing and it's like magic. It squeaks jumps, runs and hides. Play lasts for a few minutes, then the wonderful thing goes back inside the cupboard.

'We'll play again tonight Sweetie. No time now…but I have a birthday treat for you.' She scoops the best ever food into my dish.

'Tuna for you, Treasure.'

The yummy food goes too fast. I lick my lips and find a warm place in the sun to sleep…and sleep.

Day Two

I'm on the Human's big bed. It's warm here and I snuggle into the blanket. Sunlight crawls under the curtain. A big happy sigh! I lick one paw and then the other. Woooo! Woooo! …a loud, buzzing thing…such a lot of noise it makes! The Humans move quickly and their eyes open wide. His hand shoots out to kill the noise.

'Wake up!' He mutters, but puts his head back under the covers.

She yawns, stretches her arm towards me and whispers 'Come to me Sebastian, my precious'. With one grab I'm underneath and next to her warmth. She strokes my fur and talks to me softly saying. 'My best boy!'

My eyes close. I sniff her scent, always strongest before her hot, wet shower. A gentle pat, She moves me away and climbs out of bed. Pity, but heaven doesn't last long in my house.

Everything is fast and busy in the kitchen. He puts down my breakfast in a bowl filled with the hard little bits I like. Then they rush from room to room and shout. They pick up papers, bags and coats. The front door bangs and they are gone. My house is quiet now, and I can hear my purr. If only they both had a long stretch every morning, or a roll on the carpet and a yawn, they wouldn't rush so much.

I must check my house now - room by room, corner by corner and every door. I rub here and then there, to leave my mark. All is safe, but I shiver in the cold. Back to the big bed, under the covers on her side with her scent. His smell is too strong.

I wake and go to their shower to pee. What they don't see they don't know. Then I run to the other end of the house and put my head through the special door to my garden. *Whooossskssss!* Big cold drops wet my whiskers. I'm not going out today!

I go back to the kitchen for a nibble. There's no one to play with and nothing to do. I find a warm place next to a low window for washing. My thick winter coat gets a lick all over and my soft, pink bits too. Each claw I pull out with my teeth, and clean one by one. All done like Mama taught me.

If only Jasmine was still here with me. She left me when it was cold and the trees were bare. So thin and sick she was that the Humans took her away for a few days. She came home tired with a big cut stitched across her side. She slept and slept, until her cut healed. Every morning, the Humans held her head back and made her swallow dark smelly stuff to make her better. I licked her and lay next to her to make her feel good. For a while we played again.

Then one morning, she lay next to me as cold and hard as the stones in the garden. The Humans cried and stroked her body, and cried more. Then they put her in a box and dug a hole for her under the tree. I watched them put the box in the hole and cover it with soil, and place sweet pink flowers on top of it. So much crying that day! I couldn't stop…but no one can see when a cat cries.

The big garden is closed in with wire. The Humans won't let me visit Jasmine's grave in the big garden, but I can see it. I could still smell her while she became part of the earth. Then one day after the rain, the sun came out shining so brightly. That's when she crossed over the rainbow of many colours.

Day Three

I miss Jasmine so much. I will never forget her meow. If the sun is shining and I wait near her basket, sometimes she visits. Then I can see her again in all her beauty. She turns her head towards me, purrs loudly and then she leaves. I go there now. I wait and wait, but Jasmine doesn't visit me today and I feel sad.

Day Four

My best time is at night after my food. My house is warm. He lies on the couch with half-closed eyes in front of the big, noisy colour box. His hand strokes my head. I wait until She finishes banging in the kitchen. Then I leave him and jump onto her lap. That's where I belong. She makes sweet kitten noises and purring sounds, tickles my tummy, and tells me how much she loves me. I love her too.

Cuddling close, I sleep.

My Humans are laughing loudly at something on the colour box and they wake me. They hold each other's hands. Their faces touch and they lie together. There is no place for me now.

'Me, me me, *meeooooow, meeeeow*!' I call.

'Good night Sweetie,' She says, and bends to stroke me from head to tail. They kill the noise box and go to the big bed. I wait outside their room until they purr as they sleep. Then I jump onto their warm bed, and dream of Jasmine.

Day Five

My Humans are sleeping and sleeping. I am hungry, so I touch her face with my paw to wake her, but she doesn't move. I jump on her. She smiles and goes back to sleep. I lie next to her and wait. Then I leave and follow the sun. My Humans are in the bedroom for a long time. Both come out smelling of sweet flowers. Slowly she goes to the kitchen.

I follow her. *Meow, Meow*! I stare at her, purr loudly, and wait next to the food cupboard.

She understands.

'Yes, Precious, you're hungry!'

She pours food into my bowl and gives me clean water.

I hear her eating, "Chomp, chomp." Maybe she'll give me a little or drop something on the floor.

A little food falls but I don't like it.

I sit near the front door and wait for the sound of my Humans coming home. She arrives early, but doesn't stop to stroke my head or go to the kitchen to eat and drink. Instead she rushes to the bedroom. Her voice is quiet and tired. Soon She is in the big bed under the covers. I jump up next to her. She snuggles up to me and falls asleep.

He comes home. His big feet make a loud noise in his black shoes, but he tries not to wake her. He kisses her head.

'She's tired, so don't wake her!' he says to me. He doesn't realise that I understand.

I sleep next to her all night. He moves around, kicks and makes noises as She sleeps. In the morning, She opens her eyes and sees me next to her. She strokes me and says, 'You've been with me all night, Sweetie. You know how tired I was last night, don't you... but I feel great now.'

I purr and stare at her so hard that she knows I understand. She gets out of bed and I follow her to the kitchen. Perhaps today She will give me something tasty for breakfast.

His feet walk loudly to the kitchen. He eats too...and pushes me away from the table. 'Go away, cat,' He says. He had better learn not to do that!

A week later

I don't feel like writing today. It's a sunny day and I'm going into the garden. No time for writing...I'm lazy and writing interferes with my sleep. It might be a good idea to stop writing for a while.

One month later

I haven't written in my diary for a long time, and I don't feel like writing in my diary today either. On my next birthday I might write again.

I still miss beautiful Jasmine. Her scent has left the house now, but I will always love her and her meow will never leave me. Poor Jasmine, she was sick and in pain, but her time had come to rest forever. I hope she is comfortable now, in a happy place, with a soft, warm basket, and that she has plenty of tuna and chicken to eat.

Remembering the Tree of Life

Jacqui threw her satchel on the chair and ran to her grandmother. 'Gran, Gran…look. I got three elephant stamps and two gold stars at school today,' the five-year-old said, thrusting an exercise book onto her grandmother's lap.

The old woman rolled up her knitting carefully in a silk scarf and placed it on the table. 'Come and let me give you a big hug.'

Jacqui freed herself from the grey jumper and purple woolen skirt. Her grandmother's energetic hugs sometimes left her breathless. She sat on the leather ottoman, her grandmother used for lifting her swollen legs, and waited for her grandmother to speak. At this time of day, she enjoyed listening to her grandmother's stories about fairies and goblins, or tales about her life in the land over the sea where she was born.

'I have something special to give to you today,' the old woman said. Delving into her sewing box, she withdrew a small package of blue, floral paper tied together loosely with a silver ribbon. She untied the ribbon slowly and lovingly, parting the leaves of paper to show her granddaughter a square of embroidery. She smoothed it out on her lap. The piece of cream cotton was embroidered with satiny colours caught in delicate stitches that glowed.

'It took me a very long time to make this for you to keep. It took so long that I almost gave up, but thank goodness I didn't,' the old woman said. 'I love you, and it was worthwhile doing.'

'A fat tree with lots of leaves and fruit,' Jacqui said with a disappointed sigh. She was hoping for something more exciting.

'Look at the pears, Jacqui. There are so many of them and they're golden.'

'Yes Gran.' Jacqui fidgeted restlessly with the buttons of her shirt, waiting for her grandmother to give her an explanation.

186

'It's the Tree of Life, my darling. We all have a tree like that inside ourselves. It starts off small like the young trees your dad plants in the garden. If the tree is cared for, it grows tall and develops strong branches and healthy leaves. It takes a lot of work to care for a tree. A tree may take longer than others to produce fruit and need a bit more help, a little more water, or perhaps some sunlight, but if we put in the effort, eventually it will produce large, shiny, sweet fruit.' Her grandmother kissed her again. 'I'm giving you a golden pear for doing so well at school today.'

'But Gran, I haven't got a tree…so I can't eat the pear.'

'I know this is hard for you to understand now Jacqui darling, but you will later. Keep this gift in your drawer as gift from your Gran,' the old woman said, rolling up the cream linen square in the blue paper.

Jacqui stood on her toes, kissed her grandmother's lined cheek, took the gift and raced off. Later she placed it in her underwear drawer.

Twelve years later, Jacqui was at university in her first year of pharmacy studies. She found the course difficult and the number of assignments demanding. She was trying her best, but so far her marks for practical assignments were merely satisfactory, and she didn't know how to improve.

One afternoon, she returned from university disheartened after another low mark for her assignment.

Perhaps I'm not suited to the course, or I haven't got what it takes.

She looked at the photograph of her grandmother, who had died five years earlier, and felt an unbearable longing to talk to her.

I wish Gran was with me now, she'd know how to help me, what to do. She had a long list of remedies for most ailments of the spirit and the body.

As she thought of the times they had spent together, she suddenly remembered the blue, floral parcel that still lay unopened in her underwear drawer.

The ribbon broke easily in her eagerness to touch something that had been made by her grandmother. She tore away the blue paper, placed the cream square on her bedspread, stroked it and then took a step back to look at it. It was not the boring image she remembered, but an exquisitely stitched, coppery tree with vibrant, green leaves and full, golden pears. She stared at it for some time.

No wonder it had taken Gran so long to make. Now I understand. My tree is dry, bare of fruit and without leaves.

She sobbed, her tears running down her face, wetting her tee shirt.

Later that day, she thought about the story her grandmother had told her about the pears on the tree that grew inside us all.

Gran said I'd have to care for the tree if the pears were to grow and be golden, and it wasn't always easy. I'm trying but I'm impatient. I scored high grades at math, science and chemistry at school. Perhaps I'm not working hard enough or missing something.

'*Keep working hard and don't give up,*' *she heard her grandmother telling her.*

I'll speak to my tutors tomorrow and ask for help.

Growth & Learning

The Magic of Uluru

Luck can change a life, and I can happily say it changed mine. My name is Rosie. I am an Aborigine. I was born in the Northern Territory of Australia, near the base of our great rock, Uluru. When I was three-years-old my mother died. I have two older sisters and two younger brothers. Dad couldn't look after us after mum died, and we were split up. I think I was the luckiest one, because Auntie Maud and Uncle Thomas took me in. They were kind and treated me like one of their own daughters. They had five children of their own and called me number six. I had a happy childhood, and I saw my brothers and sisters often, as we lived close to each other.

From the age of about five, I enjoyed kicking balls with the boys, while other girls played with dolls. I became good at kicking and "headers" too. The quicker I moved the ball around to score goals, the more people laughed at me, "a girl playing soccer". By the time I was in my teens, I played soccer with a group of girls. There were a few other girl teams in the area and we played against each other regularly.

This is where luck entered my life. One weekend, three girls who played soccer in Sydney visited Uluru. The girls were all blonde, tanned and pretty. They had heard that we were playing soccer and made a special trip to our village to watch us play. My team, the Rockers, gave them the entertainment they were after. They shouted for us, and me in particular. I scored four goals and we won.

After the game, one of the visitors who said her name was Sam, short for Samantha, came to talk to me. She said good things about my game, and I was thrilled. I had no idea that they were scouts for their own team. When she asked if I'd ever thought of playing soccer in Sydney, I was so shocked by her interest in me that I hardly said a thing. When she was about to leave we exchanged names and email addresses. She waved and said, 'You'll be hearing from me soon.'

I had forgotten about the girl's visit when I received an email from Sam. She asked if I would be interested in coming to Sydney to join their team. A huge surprise! What an opportunity for a girl like me from the Northern Territory! Of course I was interested, but I didn't want to appear too keen. I made myself wait two days before replying. We had a long talk on the phone, and she told me all about the team. They played other women soccer teams all over Australia, and sometimes even overseas. She explained that if I wanted join them they would find me accommodation and pay me enough to live on. All the terms and conditions would be in a contract that she would send me, and I'd have to sign it.

My aunties and cousins were excited when I told them about Sam's offer. When the contract arrived, they said they would jump at an opportunity like that, but that I should ask a lawyer to check the contract before signing. The biggest problem was finding a lawyer. Finally, I went to the courthouse. I hated anything to do with courts and police, but I had no choice. The lawyer at the court was helpful. She said that the contract wasn't the best one she'd seen, the money they were offering was a bit mean, but they couldn't force me to stay if I wasn't happy, and wanted to come home after the trial period of three months.

I felt wobbly inside about leaving home. I hadn't even been as far as Darwin, and I was scared. In spite of my fears, I signed the papers and sent them back. I was absolutely terrified when I realised what I had done. What if I wasn't as good at soccer as they thought, or if I didn't fit in with the others. There was no way out now. I had to go.

My auntie reminded me that we had family in Sydney to contact. People told me to expect cooler weather there and to take some warm clothes along. I had two old jumpers and packed them in my suitcase with my few clothes and my photos. My cousin Danny drove me to the bus that went to the airport in Darwin.

All I could think of during the car ride was how scared I was of flying. But the plane trip was lovely and being in the clouds was like a dream. Sam and another girl were waiting for me at the Sydney airport. As they drove I couldn't even speak from shock. The city was even more spread out than I imagined, and the air was thick, but they were kind to me. They took me for a meal and then to the place where I would stay. It was a small room with a television, bed, bathroom and tiny kitchen, clean and big enough for me. When I unpacked, they complained that I didn't bring the correct clothes for the weather. They took me shopping and between them they paid for running shoes, socks, a jumper and a track suit. I didn't know what to say, or how to thank them. I thought that they must've wanted me to join the team badly, or they wouldn't have gone to so much expense.

The girls gave me money for the month. Once they left, I explored the area, found my way around to the cheaper shops, and bought some food. When I was introduced to the team, I found that there was an Indian girl and a Chinese one, but I was the only Aboriginal. We practiced every day and it was fun. The players were good, but I could hold my own. I was still in the trial period, and the team players seemed happy with me. I missed home and had trouble sleeping without the usual sounds of the night. In my room I heard mainly traffic noises. Phoning home every week and hearing my family's voices kept me going.

The money they gave me seemed a lot at first, but it went quickly on food and bus fare. Everything in the city cost such a lot. I didn't realise how expensive a lettuce or an orange would be in the city. The girls in the team invited me to join them for drinks and coffee after practice, but I didn't go. I didn't feel one of them yet, even though I was a member of the team. I knew I should've made more of an effort.

Around that time, I remembered that I had the phone numbers of family in Sydney. When I phoned they didn't know who I was at first, but they worked it out and said they were pleased that I had contacted them. One Sunday, they picked me up in a big car. They drove me to their double storey home in an attractive suburb with neat houses and gardens. They looked like family with the same shaped nose as mine and talked like the rest of us back home. That made me feel good. They welcomed me and we talked a lot, but they lived such a long way from my little apartment, that I knew that I wouldn't see them often.

The three months trial passed and I was accepted as a full team member. But I still felt that I didn't belong. It wasn't true of course, but I thought of myself as an extra, recruited just to score goals. Most of the girls told me I played well, but I knew I could do better. Being away from home made me less motivated. Until then, I hadn't played a match against an opposing team.

When I heard the news that I would be playing against another team the following weekend I was excited, but afraid of letting my own team down. Back home I was the most popular player on the ground, but when I played my first match in Sydney there would be no one from home calling out my name, encouraging me to do my best. I had been given a wonderful opportunity and I knew it, but I was finding motivating myself difficult.

For the first time since I left home, I took out my photos of my family and friends with Uluru dominating the background. That night I told myself, 'Uluru is more striking than the Sydney Bridge that everyone raves about. The great rock is bold and strong and it has withstood all kinds of weather. I have the dust of the great, red rock in my heart and I am not alone.'

I felt more enthusiastic and more confident about playing. I had survived the death of my parents, and become strong. I could do it, but if I was to play at my best, I knew I had to reach out to the other girls in my team. That connection was crucial. They had tried their best, done everything to welcome me, but I hadn't been friendly and responded. It was up to me now.

As I became more optimistic about my performance, I ran daily and practised with the team during the week. My show of friendliness towards the girls made a difference, and they smiled at me more. I felt less alone.

On the day of the match, Janice, one of the older team members came to talk to me. 'I have a few aboriginal friends who like soccer, but play Rugby League. Maybe you've seen some of them on television. I told them what a great player you are, and they were thrilled that you are playing with us today. They'll be here to support the team…just thought you'd like to know.'

I gave Janice a hug. 'Thank you…that's great…but I hope I won't disappoint them or the team.'

'You won't, I'm certain of that!'

We were playing a top team and when we ran onto the field I was nervous, but I told myself that the rock in me would not let me down. We played hard and were passing and kicking well, but by half-time we were two points down.

'Come on, come on…you can do it,' I told myself.

Well, I did it, and scored two goals. Sam scored two as well. We won and we were ecstatic. There were hugs all around. After the game, Janice introduced me to the aboriginal guys and their girlfriends, who had come to support us. I recognised some of them from matches on television. I was thrilled when they invited me to join them for dinner the following night.

As we talked, we found that we had family and friends in common. We laughed together and enjoyed the meal. It was the start of close friendships. Within months, I was more used to living in Sydney. I played well and enjoyed belonging to a team, and a new community. There were more matches planned for me, and an increase in salary. I was able to save a little each month to visit my family and see the Great Rock again.

Search for Meaning

Each day, Ravi examined his face for tell-tale signs of aging. From the time he turned forty-five, staying young was almost an obsession. He dieted, jogged daily and took mega doses of vitamins to maintain his health and youthful appearance. The city's best barber styled his hair, and he wore clothing that made him appear modern and stylish. No matter how young he looked for his age, he was dissatisfied.

During the past year, his job as a clerk of the court had become boring when previously it had been a challenge. To escape his rising dissatisfaction, he threw himself into social engagements, but he did not enjoy himself as before. He bought a fast car, but the pleasure he experienced racing on the freeway didn't last. Finally, he admitted to himself that he was searching for more in life. What that "more" was, he had no idea.

He pondered endlessly on the meaning of life - his life. He sought answers in his religion. When he was unable to find help from holy men, he visited sages, clairvoyants and spiritualists, but still his quest drew no satisfaction. Was there an answer he wondered, as his life became more mundane and dissatisfying?

After many months, he decided to extend his quest to India, the land of his birth. Everyone he knew who went to India returned with newfound spiritual energy. Hopefully, a visit to his ancestral home would provide the solutions he sought.

Within a few weeks he left for New Delhi. He was confronted with masses of people, noise, traffic congestion and extreme poverty. As there were several spiritually significant sites to visit, he joined a tour. The grace and haunting beauty of the Taj Mahal didn't stir him as it would have years before. He wasn't inspired deeply by ancient temples either. He flew on to Varanasi, the pilgrimage centre along the banks of the sacred Ganges River, where many others like him were on a quest for spiritual enlightenment. There he saw holy men covered in mud and ash, but their years of ritual self-sacrifice and discipline through all seasons and weather, was difficult for him to appreciate. Many pilgrims dressed in white bathed at the steps of the Ganges. Ravi saw only a filthy and polluted river with disintegrating steps and pathways, and it did not give him the connection he had anticipated.

He traveled further to the tea plantations in Darjeeling, where he had lived with his family as a young boy. The breathtaking views of the plantations with the mountain range in the background brought a lump to his throat, but the rambling old house, once his home, had been replaced by new, modern apartments. He combed the area for relatives and friends, but found that they had moved on. Dissatisfied and frustrated by his inability to satisfy his expectations, he returned home.

Back home, Ravi resumed his daily routine. When he learned that his cousin Nandapal was seriously ill and in hospital he was shocked. He and Nandapal had played together as children. A close bond existed between them, even though as adults they rarely saw each other. Armed with fruit and flowers, he visited his cousin. He found Nandapal connected to a drip, his ravaged body had shrunk and his face was pale. Ravi tried hard to lift his cousin's spirits with stories about his trip to India, but Nandapal was too ill to listen.

Each night after work, Ravi sat at his cousin's bedside. He read to him and tried to tempt his cousin's meagre appetite with delicacies. As Nandapal's illness progressed almost all his energy left him. Both men knew that death was near, yet they were closer than ever. When Nandapal died he was cremated a few days later according to religious ritual. Ravi followed all the memorial ceremonies for Nandapal. He felt the loss of his cousin intensely.

Weeks later, Ravi was thinking of Nandapal, when he realised how much he had loved his cousin. His care for his cousin was the first time since childhood that he had genuinely given of himself to anyone. He came to the conclusion that at work and socially he had been self-involved and taken from others, but not offered anything in return. The visit to India had provided none of the answers he'd sought, as he'd been closed to the experience.

Gradually Ravi changed. He no longer cared about wearing the most fashionable clothing and portraying a youthful image. He followed a more moderate regime of exercise and diet. As he became interested in reading, music and meditation for inner enrichment, his days were more serene and predictable. At court he tried to support people who felt overwhelmed by the complexities of the legal system, and provided them with the information they needed. His work day became more fulfilling.

'Perhaps there aren't any answers to my questions,' he told himself. 'But it doesn't seem as important now.'

The Cloud Spinner

Felicity eased herself into her seat in the packed airplane. As the plane took off she listened to the hum of the engine and felt a surge of excitement. This was the holiday she had looked forward to for so long. At last she was on her way. The final rush before she left had been exhausting. Everything at work had to be left tidy and easy for others to follow. A project she had been working on needed to be completed and clients notified of her absence from the office. She was a person who tried very hard to do things well, and her colleagues fondly called her a perfectionist.

Though Felicity was an attractive thirty-year-old, she had a meagre social life and no boyfriend. A broken relationship with a school sweetheart had hit her hard, and she avoided dating the many men who approached her. She went out only occasionally and instead threw herself into her work.

She adjusted her seat into a more comfortable position, smoothed down the creases in her skirt, and picked off a hair from her jacket. Through a cabin window she looked out onto an endless vista of blue, lacey clouds. Absorbed by the myriad of moving patterns in the sky, she began to drift, floating as freely as the clouds.

A woman dressed in a white, silky robe sat at a wheel spinning perfectly round clouds. Her forehead was wrinkled in concentration, and her jaw set determinedly. To keep up her pace, the spinner worked fast. Occasionally she smiled, as she watched the spheres carried out into the distance.

A sudden wind changed her clouds, making them disintegrate into mist. As the wind swirled fiercely, the sky darkened. The spinner's face was etched in disappointment. She spun the balls frantically in an attempt to fill the sky, but the heavy, grey blanket swallowed them. With the first shower, she threw her hands up in despair, packed up her spinning wheel and disappeared.

A sudden air pocket woke Jessica. She tightened the seatbelt and smiled to herself. 'If I had spun the clouds, I'd like perfect shapes too. On this holiday I'll try to ease up a bit and enjoy myself, or my life will drift away.'

The Bully

I was pleased with myself for pulling off a lucrative overseas deal after long and intense negotiation. Naturally, the company director was delighted too. The long hours of work exhausted me and I decided to take a day off. After sleeping until noon, I went shopping. A gift to myself was a new winter coat, and I bought flowers for my love, Bella, as well. Loaded with parcels, I made my way to Target for underwear. As far back as I can remember, all my underwear was purchased at Target. I was in the pay queue, when an uneasy prickly sensation at the back of my neck alerted me that someone was staring at me. As I turned around, a man lowered his eyes.

'Next,' the checkout guy called.

I paid and looked back, but the man had disappeared. As I walked out of the store he was waiting for me.

'Greg Harrison?' He asked uncertainly.

'That's me,' I replied, and looked at him – stubble on a rough sunburnt skin, greying hair that needed a trim, and he supported himself on a walking stick. His face was familiar, but right then I couldn't place him.

'Terry Lawler from Station Street High,' he said.

At first the name meant nothing to me, and then it hit me, "Terry the Tormentor". Oh, yes, I remember you!'

'I know… I made your life a misery at school, so I guess you remember me,' he mumbled, shuffling as he shifted his stick. 'I haven't come across anyone from school for ages.'

I shrugged. I had no desire to have a conversation with someone I had hated, even if it was twenty-five years ago.

'You're looking good these days,' he said as he gave me the once over.

He looked dreadfully pale and his once hefty frame had shrunk. My face must've revealed my displeasure at being in his company. 'Interesting to bump into you Terry,' I said, beginning to walk away.

Terry lifted his free hand to stop me. 'Please don't go... yet.' He moved his stick again. 'I'm sorry...about what happened at school.'

'It toughened me up for stuff later.' I replied in a sarcastic tone.

'I wish I could say I was tough now,' he said with a grimace. 'I'm not doing too well...an accident at work.'

'Oh, I'm sorry.' I saw the pain in his grey eyes for the first time.

He nodded. 'It's the way it goes sometimes in construction.'

'Yep...very dangerous work.'

'You know, sometimes I think about the monster I was back in those days, and I feel bad about it. Maybe I'm getting paid back now.'

'That's not the way, to think Terry. No one deserves what you must be going through.'

'It's good of you to say that.' He gulped, and looked away.

The man before me was nothing like the Terry who had terrified me at school, waiting for me with his thugs each morning outside the gates. I remembered them hitting and punching me, calling me a four-eyed toad, and throwing my glasses in the dirt. Once they even broke them. Back then, I lived in fear that he or one of his mates would jump out from behind a pillar or wall to attack me.

Terry leant heavily on his stick and cursed. 'I'll have to sit down soon...or fall down.' He looked about for somewhere to rest.

Behaving decently is the least I can do for any human being who is suffering, I told myself.

'Let's go over there,' I said pointing to a coffee shop cross the mall.'

We ordered coffee and talked, recalling names of our fellow classmates and teachers, and laughed over some of our school exploits. The way we locked hated Mr. Burnside in the toilet and hid Mrs. Goldstein's teaching notes, so that she went crazy hunting for them made us giggle like kids. Once we had exhausted most of our memories of school, I asked about the injury to his leg.

'I'm an electrician and work on construction sites. Seven months ago I was up on a high scaffold installing electricity when I fell. My employers wanted the building completed in a hurry... before the end of the year. In our rush there were three of us on the scaffold when the rules stated clearly that there should've only been one. It was stupid and my fault. I was the most experienced person there. I should've been more careful. The structure gave way and we all fell. I was lucky to fall on sand, but I broke my pelvis and had fractures in my left leg. The other two had worse injuries, but they are recovering. After a long spell in a hospital, I was sent to rehabilitation. I've been home for a month now, but still have to attend as an outpatient. They reckon I'll heal, but no more high rise buildings for me.'

'Nasty, but at least you're recovering,' I said.

We were both silent. I was thinking of leaving, when Terry's expression changed. He stared into the distance and his mouth quivered. 'Maybe I should tell you a bit about my home life when I was a kid. It doesn't excuse my behavior back at school, but it explains a few things.'

'OK,' I said, with a slight shrug.

'I was the oldest of three brothers. We didn't have much in those days, but both mum and dad worked, so there was always enough food on the table. The best part was that they were away all day and apart from looking out for the younger ones, I could do as I liked,' he said, sipping his coffee. 'It wasn't the best thing for a young kid. I got myself mixed up with a street gang stealing from shops, smoking grass and sometimes selling it. When one of them was caught by the cops, I got out…and just in time, I reckon.'

He looked serious when he began to talk about his parents. 'Dad liked the booze. When he'd had too much, which happened regularly, he would take it out on my mum, hitting her and calling her filthy names. When I tried to protect her from him, I'd end up with a thrashing. There was nothing I could do to change things, and I can see now how scared and angry I was then.'

I've always known that I was fortunate to have loving parents and a stable home life. I understood now that Terry had learned from watching his Dad, and he knew how power over us felt. He was too young to deal with his anger, and took it out on us kids. In many ways I guess, he was as much a victim as I and the others he preyed on were. In spite of all that he went through as a child, I wasn't going to tell him that it was alright to have made my school life hell.

He had changed for the better, but I wasn't ready to tell him my own story - that I had been injured in a skiing accident five years ago, that the doctors told me I'd be in a wheelchair for the rest of my life. But, that I fought hard through painful exercise and made it back on my feet. I would save telling him my story if we met another time.

I stood to retrieve my parcels. 'I've got to get going.'

'It's been good to talk,' he said, as he battled to grab his stick and balance.

I helped him up and once he was standing I handed him my business card. 'Give me a call Terry, and maybe we can meet sometime for a drink or coffee after work.'

'Will do…and thanks,' he said.

I knew we'd never be friends, but the least I could do was to be there for him. He badly needed to talk to someone.

Learning

Winning isn't Everything

It was the despondent way Geoff walked into the café that told me that something was wrong. I had known him since childhood days, and we had kept up our friendship. A few times a year we met for a quick lunch.

'Let's sit outside.....I've got to have a smoke and get some coffee,' he said, as we moved into the sharp air. He sighed. 'What a week...... major hassles at work.'

He didn't give me time to reply.

'Since I saw you last I was upgraded to National Manager.' He put his hand up to still my congratulations. 'But I've had nothing but trouble. I mucked up a massive deal that could've increased our profits. Sure I tried to smooth it over, but in the end I will have to leave it to the CEO to sort out.'

Though I tried to lift Geoff's mood, he left as stressed as he'd arrived.

When we met again six weeks later, I was surprised by the change in him.

'Things have picked up. I spent a week away with friends in the country, and the break did me good. It helped me to think more clearly. I've lots to tell you.'

'Let's hear it,' I said. I could tell there wouldn't be time for any of my news that day.

'I took a long walk. I was admiring the maples with their flaming leaves, when I remembered an earlier incident one autumn. I must've been about sixteen at the time. I was a good runner at school and I was chosen for the state running team. It was a huge honour. My best race was the 400 metres hurdle. It was important for me to win. I dreaded failure, and the trophy meant a lot to mum too. She followed all my races and displayed my cups on the mantelpiece.'

'Yes, I remember coming into your house with all the shining silverware gleaming. She must've cleaned it all till it shone.' I smiled at the memory.

'Those were the days,' he said with a grin.

He continued his story. 'There were months of practice. In the week before the race, I surprised myself by surpassing my personal best. My hopes rose and I expected a lot from myself. But, the closer I thought I was to winning, the more I had to lose if I failed.

'On the day of the race, I was pumped up and ready to go. From the minute I left the starting block I was ahead. Then, I increased my speed and kept a steady pace, clearing the hurdles and gaining all the time. I was ahead of the rest, when I heard a cry. I looked back. My mate Ivan had collapsed on the second last hurdle. I remember stopping for a moment and hesitating. Then I put all thoughts of winning aside, and ran back to help him. He was in pain and had hurt his ankle. Together we hobbled to the finish line with loud cheers from the crowd. I hadn't failed at all.

'Remembering that incident made me realise that my mistake at work probably wasn't as serious as I thought. As usual, I was concentrating on winning, on the financial gains the company could make. I had pushed the deal through too hard and too fast. I was expecting to score every time.'

'So what happened,' I asked.

'Once I was back at work we had a management meeting. I apologised for the loss of business and profit loss. The other members of the team looked at me surprised. Robert, the CEO laughed. He said that didn't I know it wasn't my fault. Our parent company overseas supplied the client with the wrong product. No wonder we lost the deal.'

'That was unexpected,' I said.

'Well, I have put the episode down to experience. At least I have learnt to think more logically and not to jump to conclusions,' he said with a wry smile. 'In our next meeting I'm going to suggest that we develop a new, analytical program to help us work much more closely with the parent company overseas to prevent this happening again.'

I nodded and smiled. I was pleased for him. I'd have to tell him about our plans for a new house another time. Our lunch break was over.

Vera's Recovery

My name is Vera. I am seventy-four, and I have lived in Rosedale Mansions for the last fifty years. My apartment is old, but comfortable with a magnificent view of the sea. It couldn't be more convenient, being close to the shops and to both the train and trams. The rooms are large with high rose ceilings. My grandmother's display cabinet which graces half a wall is filled to capacity with my collections - cats, owls, and of course there are pottery and glass ornaments as well. The walls are covered with paintings and etchings that belonged to my parents and grandparents, and some paintings I couldn't resist buying.

I was asked, but I chose not to marry. I have definite views on most things, and I was far too independent to bend to the bonds of marriage. However, I was rarely short of male company as a young woman. There were lonely moments with touches of regret for having no children and grandchildren, but there were many advantages of being single with no responsibilities apart from work constraints. I relished indulging my whims and doing as I wished without anyone asking questions. During the Christmas break I travelled both locally and overseas to unusual places every year. I was impulsive and adventurous then, and probably foolhardy enough to go "white water rafting", parachuting from a plane and deep sea diving.

As a child, I'd thought it normal that my father didn't work, and that we ate beans on toast for dinner when food parcels from the government ran out. My mother took in ironing, and was so busy that she was unaware that I hung out on the beach with the boys most afternoons. School and girlie talk bored me, but surfing was exciting. I was good at it too. In senior school my grades dropped so low that that my teachers didn't even bother to suggest that I apply for a scholarship to finish my schooling, and then study further. 'Leave school when you're sixteen and go to trade school,' my class teacher said. I didn't have a choice. I had to leave school. My family needed any money I could earn to feed my brothers and sister.

I can remember clearly the day I began working at Morrison's, an upmarket bakery. Soon I learned to bake a wide variety of breads and cakes. Though I formed friendships and enjoyed the work, I was ambitious. I wanted more, and began to save a small amount of my wages. When I was twenty-five, I opened my own modest bakery and café. Within a short while, locals and visitors came to my shop.

Shortly after I turned sixty-six, I had a virus that developed into a serious form of pneumonia, and kept me in hospital for six weeks. I don't remember much of what happened in hospital, apart from the discomfort of tubes that stopped me from talking, having oxygen, and a line of drips that provided antibiotics. Once I improved, the tubes were removed. The doctor told me that I was extremely lucky to have survived. He warned me not to tire myself too much in future or... He didn't finish the sentence.

The shock of my brush with death was frightening, and it changed me. I left hospital feeling weak and afraid for the first time. I retired from work. Luckily my shop sold at an excellent price. But retirement didn't make me happy. In my worried mood, I withdrew from my friends and former activities. For the next year and a half my life was quiet and structured. The predictability of routine made me feel safe. Of course I knew that none of us can control unexpected events in our lives, but it helped me to imagine that I could.

Each morning, I continued to rise early to bake breads, croissants and muffins for a homeless shelter and a women's refuge in the area. Since my illness, the baking that had once come easily, exhausted me, but I rested and then persevered.

Baking was one of the things I could do to make life more pleasant for people who were struggling like I once did. After the baked goods were collected, I walked along the beachfront. At first, I was too weak to keep going for more than ten minutes before flopping exhausted on the beach. Gradually my stamina improved until I could walk for an hour. In all its moods, the sea calmed me. People I passed on the beach nodded in greeting and smiled. Then, that was all the contact I wanted. My afternoons were organized too. I was home for a small lunch, and then I had a daily nap. There was shopping to do later if I wasn't too tired. At night I watched a little television.

Somehow, my ordered life helped me to recover. I had been tough on myself since childhood. If I promised myself I would do something, I stuck to it. It was a pity I hadn't felt strongly about achieving high grades at school.

As I became stronger, the protective structure I had created, felt like a cage. My fears had left me, but I was lonely and longed for the stimulation of new activities. When I tried to contact old friends, some were sickly, others had moved to live with their children, or were in special accommodation homes. The few still living in the area had found new friends, or were annoyed that I had disappeared without a word.

Three women in the apartment building were friendly. They walked on the beach together in the morning, and instead of walking alone, I joined them. Occasionally, I invited my new friends for afternoon tea. It was my pleasure to make them cakes and cookies while we chatted animatedly about their lives and grandchildren. I had always been secretive and I didn't talk about my past. They wouldn't have believed that I'd had more boyfriends than they'd had in their dreams.

Thanks to their encouragement, I enrolled for an art course at the local senior centre. I was surprised that I could paint fairly well. There hadn't been time for a hobby while I worked. Now I enjoyed being creative.

It didn't take me long to realise that I was the only person in my art group who didn't understand how to use a computer. Technology was everywhere, but I had managed my life without a computer or smart phone. I decided to join a beginners computer group. Learning this new skill was surprisingly difficult, and I wondered how most people in the world were able to master it.

Raynor who lived next door, owned a computer. She kindly allowed me to try out my new skills. One afternoon, while I was sending an email to a relative from her computer, her nephew Charlie visited her. He had brought his iPad along and was happily playing a game on it. The tablet he was engrossed in, caught my interest. When he demonstrated some of its functions I was overwhelmed. I was drawn to the small device that could open a new world with the touch of a few buttons.

My adventurous streak was still alive, and the image of the tablet nagged. I could afford to buy it, I told myself. I had learned how to operate a computer, so I was sure that I could transfer my skills to the tablet. During one of my visits to the shopping centre, I stopped at a store selling computers and other devices. The variety of technology amazed and confused me. With the help of a friendly salesman, I found the section displaying tablets. The salesman suggested the simplest of the tablets to operate. He pointed to young people in the store who were helping clients with their iPads. He assured me that within a week or two I would be able to use all of its functions. Impulsively I bought the iPad.

With Raynor's help, I found a technician who connected my new toy to Wi-Fi, and explained some of its basic functions. In exchange for chocolate cookies, Charlie taught me more about the tablet. I went back to the store for a few extra lessons as well. It took me longer than a week, but I learned to use my iPad and loved it. The iPad changed my life. Instead of a nap every afternoon, I logged on to the Internet. To save time and energy, I ordered my groceries online. For relaxation, I listened to music and searched for art galleries. If I wore my glasses, I could even draw on the surface of the tablet. What a delight!

Though I was reluctant to join Facebook at first, through it my life was enriched, as I resumed old friendships, some going back to my school days, and connected with relatives I barely knew.

When I recognised Fred, an ex-lover, on Facebook, I contacted him immediately. Since our affair years ago, his wife had died. Spontaneously, we resumed a friendly online relationship. There was so much to remember and to discuss. Tired of messaging each other, we decided to meet for coffee. Our friendship had not changed. We were relaxed with each other and met regularly for dinner. When Fred suggested that we take a cruise to Europe together, I jumped at the idea. I missed travelling and the cruise was the first of our adventures. Though I had visited many of the places years earlier, they had changed as I had. The best part was that there was a trip to look forward to every year.

Through my iPad I make connections with my past and learn about the constant changes in the world. I continue to bake for my charities and walk along the beach. Once again, each day is full and interesting.

A Scary Flight

I locked my car door and walked away from the airport's long term parking garage with a feeling of dread. Would I be back to claim my car in a week?

I was expected in London for company meetings. I had tried to convince my boss that my contribution would be valueless, and that the cost of my flight was a waste, but he didn't fall for it. Since childhood, I had been scared of flying and tried every way I knew to avoid it. It was the thought of being trapped, suspended in a tube with wings that might snap or fall out of the sky at any time.

For many years, I'd managed by swallowing a tranquilizer to "knock me out" through the journey, but since the horrific events of 11th September and other plane disasters, my anxiety rose. My doctor reluctantly agreed to increase my prescription. I didn't need the internet and television to alert me to the hazards of our world, my fear kept me on the lookout.

As I entered the terminal, I took several deep breaths to calm myself but it didn't work. My heart was a tom tom. At the counter I checked in my suitcase. The night before, I had struggled to close it with the selection of clothes I thought I might need in the event of weather changes.

The airport was buzzing with early morning travellers, airport officials and guards. The baggage check in queue was long and passengers were restless. Security had been stepped up since my last trip, but I liked that. The more stringent the security, the safer I felt. By the time I had passed through the magnetic arches, my stomach was a haven for butterflies. 'Keep going.... keep going,' I told myself, as I pushed myself towards the passenger waiting area. The flight was delayed only ten minutes, but the wait seemed longer.

Concentrate on others, not on yourself and you'll feel better. I had read in a magazine that being aware of the other people around me could reduce anxiety. I took a few deep breaths and surveyed the rows of people in their uncomfortable chairs. A large, Middle Eastern looking man in a creased beige suit grabbed my attention. He fiddled with the lock on his case. My fear monitor took a jolt.

Surely not...no...he couldn't be. My mind raced. *He's been through security...and I'm being totally irrational...and a bigot,* I spoke to myself firmly, but I remained unconvinced. A crisp female voice interrupted my fear fantasy with boarding instructions.

My hand luggage was tucked into the overhead locker and I was tightening my seat belt, when the man I had been staring at eased himself into the seat next to me. The butterflies inside gripped me. I made an instant decision not to take my relaxing magic pills on the flight. During this flight I had to be vigilant.

I observed his short, but luxuriant beard, tired looking olive eyes and sensual mouth. I had to admit to myself that he was handsome. He struggled to place his case under the seat, but as soon as we were airborne, he pulled it out again. As he snapped the locks I shut my eyes, my imagination conjuring disaster. Through my eyelashes I watched him select a notebook and pen and replace the case. Refusing coffee, he wrote furiously in a script I found illegible. *Evil plans, Just as well I can't read his handwriting.*

In an attempt to stem my worry, I flipped through a magazine, but the words swam and photographs of glamorous people looked more unreal than usual. I replaced the magazine in the rack, and tried to breathe slowly and relax, but I was trying too hard and it didn't work.

The flight attendant was collecting plastic coffee cups when the intercom crackled with the captain's voice. 'We have an emergency. An elderly passenger has collapsed. I would appreciate the immediate assistance of any doctors or nurses on board.'

The man next to me flung his notes and pen to the floor, reached for his case, and following a worried looking flight attendant, rushed down the aisle.

Shelter from the Storm

Conner looked at the summer sky as he wheeled his bike out of the garage. The clouds were banking up, but he figured he could manage a short ride before it rained. The spin of the wheels beneath him and the feeling of freedom after a stressful day at work was so enjoyable that he did not notice the darkening sky. Riding fast, he missed his usual turning and found himself in streets that looked unfamiliar. The large houses with abundantly flowering gardens fascinated him, and he rode further. The first drops of rain didn't bother him, but when lightening streaked the sky followed by claps of thunder, he looked for shelter. By then, the sheets of rain were almost blinding. A large building on the corner of the street seemed the most suitable place to wait out the storm. He rode through the gates and after placing his bicycle against a wall, he tugged at the double doors. They opened into an entrance foyer that looked a bit like the entrance to his church.

A door was open and he went through it. He was in an impressive place of prayer with wooden benches instead of pews, velvet curtains, a raised platform, a lit lantern, and stained glass windows. He cast his thoughts back to his classes on different religions and realised that he was in a synagogue.

A prayer book was open. Before him was Psalm 23. *The Lord is my shepherd; I shall not want. He makes me lie down in green pastures: he leads me beside the still waters.* It was one of his favourite psalms in his own prayer book. He leafed through the book, reading the English translation opposite the Hebrew letters, noticing some prayers similar in essence to those in his own prayer book.

The pounding of the rain on the roof had eased, and he was about to leave when an old, bearded man approached him. 'You've been here for a while visiting our place of prayer. Can I help you?'

'Oh…I came in to shelter from the storm. I hope that's alright,' Connor said hesitantly.

'Of course…it's fine. This is a place of prayer and shelter.'

'Yes…I know,' Connor replied.

'I'm the *shammas*…like a sexton…but the Rabbi is upstairs if you would like to talk to him.'

'No, no please don't bother him.'

Connor was looking at the ornamental cabinet with velvet curtains inside, when the old man commented. 'I think you're looking at the holy *Aron Kadesh* or Ark. It houses the *Torah Scrolls*…that contain the first five books of Moses…our law, our way of life.'

Conner nodded. 'I am enjoying the calm and peace here.'

The rain had stopped in the evening sky. The old man turned to Connor. 'You are welcome to stay a little longer, but I wiill have to lock up in a while.'

Conner thanked the old man and collected his bike. He made his way paying careful attention to the road signs and found his home easily. After a warm shower, he closed his eyes, reviving the atmosphere of calm and peace of the synagogue, and the welcoming old man. He would take more wrong turns in future.

Healing

The Wheel of Fortune

Daryl was unpredictable and unreliable at work and irritable and changeable at home. His instability threw his life into disarray, and upset other people. He dismissed his erratic behaviour as a phase that would eventually pass.

As usual, on Friday after work, Daryl went to the casino. As he swaggered into the casino, he slicked back his hair and smiled confidently. He was feeling on top of things, and in the mood for gambling. He had a look at the mass of people, the plush interior and smiled, as he grabbed a drink from a passing waitress. The pulsating pace invaded his senses. He could hardly wait to have a go.

I can feel it in my bones. Today is going to be my lucky day. I won't hold back, I'm going to give it my all.

The dazzling cave with its lights flickering hypnotically thrilled him. As he sipped his drink, he eyed an attractive, scantily dressed woman. The rows of clinking slot machines beckoned. He tried his luck and won a few dollars. The cascade of coins tinkling through the machine was a thrill, a cause to celebrate with a double whisky.

Roulette was his favourite game. The spinning wheel excited him. With a stir of almost childish delight he placed several of his chips on the table. As the tiny ball stopped at his number, adrenaline raced through him with such power that it was hard to contain his urge to shout with joy. He piled up his winnings, celebrated with another double and moved on. A patrolling muscle man watched him suspiciously.

I knew I'd win. I've got to keep going with my lucky streak.

He moved on to the blackjack tables that filled the centre aisle. The dealers in their neat uniforms stood poised for action.

Come on, come on 21.

He rubbed his hands together in anticipation. He tried to concentrate on the cards and count their values, but his mind wandered. After several games, he had lost all that he had won. The group of other players clustered around the table looked up momentarily, and then went on with their own quest. Full of hope, he worked his way down the black grotto crammed with tables and gamblers, towards the Wheel of Fortune. The name appealed to him. He was so certain that his numbers would come up, that impulsively he put down a huge sum of money hoping for a killing. The lights danced while he lost and lost again. He had been drinking heavily and felt unsteady. Flopping into a chair, he wiped his flushed face with his handkerchief. As the wheel spun and the fairy lights beckoned to him, a mixture of tiredness and alcohol overwhelmed him. He felt floaty, a sensation of being present and yet far away at the same time. Then his blurred vision sharpened.

He found himself in a functional gambling hall. The dark, voluptuous cocoon with its myriad of fairy lights had disappeared. The roulette and blackjack tables were made of a practical plastic composite now. At least the clink of gambling machines and the sound of a win with an avalanche of coins surging through the machine had not changed. There were no croupiers. They had been replaced by robots, and most of the games took place on large colourful screens. There were no cashiers either, as machines took care of all dealings. He looked around at the gamblers all dressed in similar clothing, and shrugged.

He moved to the Wheel of Fortune, picked up a few chips and threw them down. Heavens, this place is boring, he thought. A tall man next to him must've noticed his dissatisfaction and commented, 'This is 2030, you know. We're proud of our changes from the decadence earlier in the century…your time, judging by your clothes.'

'We're in 2030?' Daryl repeated, stunned. 'At least people haven't given up gambling. I'm pleased about that.'

'There are more gamblers now than before,' the man said. 'The government has tried to get rid of drugs and gambling, but given up. It's a waste of their time.' He touched Daryl's arm. 'Come, I'll show you what's happened to your world.'

Daryl followed him out of the main exit and into a street lined with shacks. He gasped at the beggars on the pavements, and the ground strewn with syringes.

'They make up about a tenth of the population...fed by the state and given free medical treatment, but it hasn't helped.' He sighed. 'Look at them! We've conquered all the old diseases like cancer, diabetes and AIDS, made progress with heart conditions using genetic engineering and nuclear medicine, but these people are our shame. If it wasn't for my wife pulling me away from drugs a few years ago, I'd be one too. I'm still an addict and can't stop gambling.'

Daryl and his new friend left the sad, ugliness of the streets and returned to the casino. When the man left to try his luck on one of the machines, Daryl sat on an uncomfortable chair.

It must've been the tinkle of glass and the loud applause accompanying a winning spin that carried Daryl back into the cave with its flickering lights. He looked around to assure himself that he really was back in the year 2017, and sighed with relief. The wheel whizzed, and he continued to play half-heartedly with the few chips in his hand. His peek at the future hadn't pleased him at all.

There were no clocks in the casino. He cursed for purposely leaving his watch at home. Picking up his remaining chips, he stumbled towards the cash desk.

'Easy now, mate...isn't it about time for you to go home?' declared a powerfully built man. 'I'll call a taxi for you.'

Daryl didn't reply, but seethed with fury.

How dare that upstart tell me what to do!

After the large amount of alcohol he had consumed, he woke with a headache, that kept him in bed for most of the next day. His exhilarated mood had left him and he felt guilty about the money he had gambled away.

'Yeah, yeah,' he answered his wife, who suggested he seek help for his drinking and gambling.

Always the gambler, he took a coin out of his pocket.

Heads I phone a help line, tails I don't. He tossed the coin into the air and it landed on tails. *Oh well, I'll see how I go over the next few months.*

Looking for Trouble

My first holiday away from home was fun in the beginning. I spent the morning, at the beach, had lazy afternoons, and was out till late at night. One night, I joined friends at a disco I hadn't been to before. We had heard good things about it and wanted to give it a try. I took care with my appearance and wore my new red, low-cut dress with high-heeled shoes.

The atmosphere and music was great. I was having a ball on the dance floor when Kevin, blond, green-eyed and handsome, caught my eye. He noticed me too and left his friends to come over for a chat. Then he bought me a drink. I didn't know a thing about him and neither did any of my friends, but I fancied him. Soon we were drinking wine and dancing. When we took a break he dipped his hand into his pocket to offer me a tablet. I refused to take it as the room was too dark to see what he was giving me.

He disappeared a few times, but between those interruptions, we danced until the early hours. He seemed to know a lot of people and waved to them. He was fun and popular, and I was enjoying myself. I had consumed a lot of alcohol, and didn't query any of his actions.

When we left the disco, we walked a few steps. Suddenly he tried to push me into an alley. The cops were parked near the entrance of the disco in an unmarked car. Luckily for me, they were there in seconds. A policeman grabbed Kevin. They searched him and found his pockets crammed with crystals that I thought could be the drug Ice. I shuddered, horrified. Was he pushing this dangerous drug? Then they looked in my handbag. I was stunned. It was packed with ecstasy tablets. Kevin must have put the tablets in my bag while I was chatting to a friend.

I began to cry. When I calmed down I realised that I couldn't do a thing about it. Not then anyway. The cops drove us to the station. I was offered a phone call, but I was scared of phoning home, especially at that time night. My parents would've freaked ,and they were too far away to do anything to help me right then. The cops held me until morning. I thought it wouldn't be long, as it was almost dawn. The small cell had a hard, narrow bed. Though I was tired and woozy from the alcohol, sleep wouldn't come. I lay there thinking how Kevin had used me and how close I had been to danger. I was furious with myself for being taken in by him.

I was nodding off at last, when I noticed a row of letters carved into the cell wall spelling the name "Janie." As I touched the letters a mist filled the cell. After a while a form defined itself. There before me stood a small, plump woman, dressed in old-fashioned prison garb.

'*Thanks for calling me up, dearie, I'm a bad old girl, but I've come to see you tonight, to help you. I was in this lock-up too. It was so miserable in here that I realised that if I didn't take control of my life, others would. I was just like you, green and taken in by good looking guys.*'

I rubbed my eyes, and shook my head hard, but her image didn't shift.

'*You can't imagine the things I did when I got out of my parent's clutches, and was in a fun mood. I drank too much and wasn't careful enough with the guys I met. I got wise later.*

'*One day when I was riding the crest of the waves, my so-called friend Nancy set me up. It's a long story, but I think she was jealous of me. I had a boyfriend and people said I was a "looker", while she was a frump and the boys didn't give her a second look. While we were trying on clothes in a shop, she stole an expensive dress. I didn't see her put it in my carry bag. Anyway, she pinned the theft on me, and I ended up in here. It's a tough world and I suppose I had to learn the hard way.'*

I shuddered, wishing she would leave, but her high-pitched voice rattled on. She waggled a fat finger at me.

'Remember to be kind to yourself and don't trust strange men. You never know what they could get up to. After all, if you don't look after yourself, who will?'

She stood on her toes, raised her round body, twirled about and then faded.

I drifted into sleep and dreamed about Kevin and the drugs. The morning clatter in the cells woke me. I had a king sized headache, but they gave me some hot coffee that helped. When Kevin was questioned, he admitted that he had put the tablets in my handbag. They charged him, but let me go.

On the bus back to the motel, I wondered about Janie. Was she a ghost, my imagination, or was I drunk and hallucinating? Whoever or whatever she was, she had come to help me. A cool wind of relief spread through me, I'd had a lucky escape from Kevin. I did not want to think about what could've happened if the cops hadn't been there when he tried to push me into the alley. All I wanted then was a shower, and to sleep in a clean and comfortable bed.

I went on lots of holidays after that one, to resorts, faraway places and camping in the bush, but this holiday had invaluable memories for me. I didn't forget Janie's old-world wisdom.

The Road to Recovery

Tony was about to open another bottle of beer, when he felt a sudden, warm heaviness on his lap. He could have sworn that sitting there contentedly was a little alien with a pale pointed face. It stared at him with its blue, slanted eyes. He was ready to push it away when he heard a deep, steady purr from the creature. It was a cat that must've crept in through the open window. Looking down at its markings, he recognised it was female Siamese, a beauty with an elegant, pale, lilac-grey body and velvety, grey tipped ears, paws and tail. He tentatively placed a hand on her head and stroked her. Her purr deepened as she snuggled up to him.

'Don't get too comfortable, you can't stay,' he said to her.

He asked neighbours if they had lost a cat, and put up notices. He became used to her around and when she wasn't claimed after a month, he kept her. The name he gave her was Ally, because he had first thought she was an alien.

Without being aware of it, Tony talked to the cat. She responded with a meow or a throaty purr.

'Another day…I might as well make the best of it,' he said to her, opening another bottle. 'One more won't hurt will it?' he said, as he tickled her tummy. When he'd had too much to drink he attempted to explain it away to Ally. 'I know I shouldn't, but I can give it up any time I like…and when I'm ready I will, but right now I need it.'

With Ally on his lap, purring as he stroked her velvety fur, he felt more at peace. Ally made herself at home the way that cats do, by sleeping on his bed as if she owned it, sitting on his lap, and on the chairs. She sniffed at the scraps of paper, greasy plates and empty bottles lying about, and lifted her paw in disdain. He muttered excuses to himself, and to her about the mess, but rarely cleaned up.

Ally spent most of her day sleeping in a warm spot. Towards evening she usually had crazy spells when she'd dash across the room and back. He was boiling the kettle for coffee one evening, when Ally jumped into a high kitchen cupboard. He heard the clink, then the smash of breaking china. Seconds later, Ally leapt down on the floor with a howl, furiously licking her bleeding paw. She seemed unhurt apart from a cut paw. He gently bandaged her foot. The next day, when her paw continued to bleed he put her in a cardboard box with a cushion at the bottom, and took her to the vet. As he expected, her front paw needed stitches. Some of his week's drinking money went to the vet, and he knew that there would be at least another consultation to check her progress. Ally had become so much part of his life, that he couldn't bear the idea of her being in pain.

A few weeks later, her paw healed and she was as active as usual. Around this time, Tony received a letter from his wife. They had been separated for two years, but he still hoped for reconciliation. Her cold, matter-of-fact words in the letter upset him. He drank to numb the pain of his longing for what might have been. In a semi-stupor, he forgot to feed Ally or leave her water.

When he recovered, he looked for Ally in all her hiding places, the linen basket, behind the curtain, and under the bed covers, but she had gone. The window she had originally come in through was open. He desperately wanted her back, but there was no sign of her. After three days of searching, he gave up, thinking he would never see her again. He blamed himself. 'If I hadn't been drunk again this wouldn't have happened. I've pushed everyone I care for away, my wife, friends and now Ally. It's all my fault.'

He punished himself by not touching a drink for two days, but had to spend the next day in bed due to withdrawal symptoms. He shook so uncontrollably that he had to have a few to settle himself down. He made one more attempt to abstain totally from drinking, but the identical symptoms made him realise he was locked into a cycle he couldn't break.

Weeks later, he was relaxing in his easy chair, when he felt a familiar heaviness in his lap. It was Ally. She was thin, her formerly shiny coat dull and matted. He opened a tin of tuna casserole and she ate hungrily. Later, while he petted her, he made up his mind to stop procrastinating.

'It's time I looked after both of us,' he said to her. 'I'm no good to you or anyone else if I keep drinking, but I can't give up the booze on my own. I'll have to ask for help.'

A local doctor booked him into a detox centre to treat his addiction. Before he left, he asked a reliable friend to look after Ally. This time he wouldn't take the chance of losing her. The period of withdrawal was awful. The physical cravings, the restlessness and the way he hurt all over made him hate alcohol and despise his weakness.

Weeks later, he returned home after his ordeal emotionally drained, his legs like jelly. Without the blunting of alcohol, his emotions were easily stirred and unpredictable. He longed for a drink to feel calmer. Though he tried to occupy himself by tidying his home, he felt agitated, and his cravings for alcohol continued. Until then, he had refused to attend an AA (Alcohol Anonymous) group as the doctors had suggested, but he was in trouble, and he knew he needed support.

'It's time for more human help,' he said to the cat while stroking her.

He attended AA meetings in his suburb regularly. Mike, a long term member of the group became his mentor and helped him as he struggled along his journey to recovery. Ally was always there to welcome him home after the meetings.

A Tough Trip

Merv cleared his throat to grab the attention of the group of school children who were given time off their lessons to hear him talk about drugs.

'I'm Merv, and I have a tough story to tell you guys about what happened to me and three of my mates, Dean, Rob, and Josh, just two years ago. At the time, we were all smoking Marijuana…Weed, and some of us were into heavier stuff. First, I'll tell you a bit about my mates.

'Dean was seventeen then, a top student and star sportsman, and leader of our group of friends. He was training and didn't smoke cigarettes, but had a little Weed with the rest of us on weekends. We were all smoking it and he didn't want to be the odd one out.

'At sixteen, Rob was a bit of a worrier. He smoked Weed whenever he could get it to calm himself down. Sport didn't interest him. He liked to listen to music while he smoked. One day he admitted that he was beginning to depend on it.

'The youngest was fifteen-year-old Josh, small for his age, sensitive and with a great sense of humour. He drew cartoons that were real likenesses, and amazing pictures of demons and dragons. We've all got one of his pictures on our walls. Josh is the smartest, most creative of the four of us. He smoked more Weed than the rest of us on a regular basis. We all knew that he was virtually an addict. We'd watch him popping Speed or Ecstasy as well as Weed, to experience that extra "buzz', especially when he was drawing or painting. Recently he told us he'd tried Ice. He said it brought out his creativity, and that it was by far the best drug he'd used so far.

'I'll tell you about myself now. I was sixteen at the time. I tried hard to look like a cool, fun guy, but I was unsure of myself. When Weed was available I'd smoke it several times during the week, but I had to be careful. My mum could smell it from down the passage. She banned it in the house, hoping that the problem would go away. I tried other drugs - downers, uppers, and E at parties, but I preferred Weed. I kept away from Ice. At night, when mum was asleep, I smoked it. Weed helped me to unwind enough to fall asleep. Yeah, I guess I was an addict.'

Merv drank some water and took a few deep breaths before continuing with his story.

'Well, this is what happened to the four of us and made us change our ways. Every Friday afternoon after school, we met under the bluestone railway bridge down the road. I bet you all know it...just three blocks from here. We fooled around and had fun, cheering and whistling like kids when a train passed overhead. It was a place where we could share the week's news, but most of all we went there to smoke Weed.

'We relied on Dean. He knew where to buy the best blend from dealers in the city. One particular week he was excited. He said that he'd scored a pure supply that came from a "special crop." It was drizzling that day and we huddled under the bridge. After a train rattled past, we cut the Weed with tobacco and rolled the mix in cigarette paper. We lit up. As each of us took a few draws there were sighs of pleasure. We went off into our own corners to enjoy the experience. We loosened up as we smoked as it was easy to discuss our feelings in a freer way than usual.

'At first we were too involved with ourselves, to notice Josh. It was Rob who pointed out that Josh looked strange. He had gone quiet, his eyes were wide and he looked scared. He didn't speak, but his hands moved around agitatedly, touching things we couldn't see. With his head tilted to one side, he listened attentively to sounds only he could hear. We all realized that Josh was having a "bad trip", but we couldn't reach him. Josh was imaginative and sometimes saw weird things when he smoked Weed, but nothing like this had ever happened before.

'Rob lifted Josh's arm, felt his fast pulse and looked concerned. "He's racing. Maybe he took something else earlier, or together with weed for a lift. You know that he's been into Ice lately." Josh's face went even paler and Dean said, "We'd better get him some help…and fast."

'Rob phoned for an ambulance. When the paramedics arrived they tried to calm Josh. Then they placed him on a stretcher and took him to a hospital in the city. We followed in a bus and waited at Emergency to find out how Josh was doing. An hour passed or more until a nurse came out to tell us that Josh was being moved to the psychiatric ward for observation.

'Josh remained in hospital after they had assessed him. Over the weekend, the three of us visited him bringing chocolates, fruit and naughty magazines to cheer him up. As we walked towards the ward, we passed Josh's parents who were leaving. They looked upset and worried. His mother stopped us. "You boys could've got Josh killed with your drug taking." Her voice was shrill with distress.

"'Come Marla, don't upset yourself. I think they realise how serious this is. No good going on about it," Josh's father said.

'We all stared at the floor, but said nothing.

'Josh looked sad and tense, sitting cross-legged on top of the bed. He was trying to stop his body shaking.

"'Thanks…thanks…mates," he said in a whispering voice that seemed disconnected to his body. He looked around and mumbled, "Sorry for all the trouble."

'We asked how he was feeling. He shrugged as he answered, "It's been Hell…the fear and the withdrawal…not out of it yet. The doc is putting me on a rehabilitation programme…and my parents are keen on me doing it…hope it helps."

'He told us that we had all been in his nightmare vision that afternoon under the bridge. We were huge, distorted and frightening. It was our eyes and voices that he thought were watching and threatening him. He admitted that he had taken Ice with Weed that afternoon. "The doc said I was lucky to come through it with all the stuff in my system, especially the Ice. Never want to see any of that stuff again. Never ever," he mumbled. The three of us, who had initially understood nothing of Josh's terrors, said our goodbyes in hushed tones. Outside the hospital, each of us expressed our horror that what had started off as a pleasant, weekly meeting under the bridge, had come to this. Josh's experience had put our own drug taking habits under the microscope.

'In the bus home, Rob spoke in a tone that betrayed his concern. "Poor guy looks awful and he's very, very sick."

'Dean said nothing for a while, and then added, "I hope that the rehab programme helps him." He looked out of the window as he talked. "We don't even know if the Weed we've been smoking has been mixed with something else. It's too dangerous…time to stop."

"'I'm through with all drugs after seeing Josh today," Rob said, "I wish I hadn't started."

'We were all silent, trying to digest our experiences, and wondering what would happen to our friend. None of us suggested meeting at the bridge again the following Friday.'

'Well, that's our story about drugs,' Merv said to the group. 'I'm at uni now studying psychology, but I do some talks about drugs to groups like this one. I need to share my experiences and hope it helps.' He looked out at the group. 'Any questions?'

The Soldier

Doug was describing his memories of his deployment to Afghanistan to a group of soldiers who were having trouble coping with Post-traumatic stress disorder (PTSD).

'I've always wanted to be a soldier. At five, I played soldier games. By nineteen, I was trained and ready to go. My first deployment was to Afghanistan. I was known as a joker then, felt ten-foot tall and totally bulletproof. I wanted to make it as sergeant soon and thought nothing could stop me.

When I arrived there, it was totally different to anything I knew. For a start, the terrain and the way that the people lived wasn't like anything I'd ever seen before. The smell of the place and lack of hygiene was an eye opener. We were there to train their army and support the civilians, but some of them were openly antagonistic to us…didn't want to know us and wanted us out of their country.

The worst part was that we didn't know who we could trust… who the real enemy was. Going on patrol I was constantly on edge, not knowing what to expect. I guess that's war for you, but I hadn't anticipated feeling so scared. Not that I breathed a word of my fear to my mates.

I was lucky. I wasn't injured, not physically, that is. It wasn't the enemies out there that got to me, but the demons inside. One particular incident stayed with me. We were in a light-armoured vehicle with my mate Baz driving. Things were going fine until were hit by an IED (improvised explosion device). Then suddenly everyone was yelling and screaming. We all scrambled out in clouds of smoke…except Baz. When we got to him, he was trapped, slumped over the wheel…dead. I still can't get his mangled body out of mind.

When I returned to Australia, I was welcomed by my family, but I felt weird…sort of detached. My wife complained, said I didn't love her. What could I say? I was dead inside…had no feelings for her or my kids, and no interest in anything. It was awful.

What happened to my mate in Afghanistan stayed with me. There weren't any specific incidents that told me I wasn't feeling right, but rather a number of jolts. One was finding out that a mate I'd played football with at school had been killed in Afghanistan. Then, when we were having dinner with friends, someone sneaked up on me to give me a hug. I didn't see her coming and I freaked. There were times when I was driving, and if a driver cut in front of me I couldn't control my anger. I wasn't sleeping much and hit the booze heavily. It was my uncle who was a Vietnam veteran who convinced me that I had a problem, and that I needed help. Some of my mates have been back to Afghanistan and to Iraq several times. They seem to be cut out for war, but I'm different.

I asked my regiment for help. I was referred to doctors and a psychologist. I had to take pills and see the psych weekly. The tablets helped a bit, but it was talking it all through that really helped.

I thought one of the things the psych wanted me to do was a bit of a laugh, but in the end it helped me most of all. She asked me to bring my phone with my photos from Afghanistan to the sessions. I had a whole lot of them, but I hadn't looked at them since coming home. Well, what we did wasn't easy. She got me to print out one picture at a time. We'd look at the picture together, talk about it, and move on to the next one. All the memories I wanted to forget came flooding back. There was one stage when it got too much for me. I didn't go back for my sessions for a month.

She rang me at home, and convinced me to keep working through the photos. It took about a year or more to go through them all. Once that was done, I felt a lot better. Then she asked me to organise the pictures and paste them into an album. She wanted me to write a bit about each photo with the names of the people and places, and anything else I could remember. I wasn't keen on doing it, but I did it to please her. She was a lovely lady. It took another few months, but the result was amazing. I came off the meds and felt better…not as good as new, but reasonably normal. I was sleeping again and not drinking much, except at meals or on occasions. I started working and had a new life.

So mates, I can tell you from my own experience, get some help if you're struggling with memories of war. You don't have to feel that way and you deserve to be helped. There are no medals for suffering.'

Gemma's Fear

Gemma was a small woman with greying hair and fine worry lines on her attractive face. Her talent was playing the piano. She started playing at five, and by sixteen she had won at least a dozen medals at different eisteddfods. Though she studied teaching after leaving school and taught history and music, she gave up her job to become a concert pianist. When she married Russel, a well-regarded tenor, she often accompanied him on the piano. With no children, music became the focus of their lives.

After Russel's early death, she walked past her piano daily, stroked its highly polished surface, but couldn't bring herself to play. It belonged to another time when she was happy. Russel had been her mainstay, and without him she was lost. She felt so vulnerable and helpless that she was afraid of leaving her house. Even the thought of leaving made her legs turn to jelly.

From her study that looked out onto the garden, she ran her home and her life. She ordered food from the supermarket online, and had it delivered. Her accountant visited if she needed him, and her doctor made home visits. All her banking was online and anything else she needed, Maria who cleaned her house, bought for her. Perhaps without all the 'home help' she may have been forced to venture out of the house.

When she received an invitation to play at the city's concert hall, she was flattered. Even if she could bring her playing to the necessary level, she was certain that she wouldn't be able to leave her house, but the idea of playing on stage again was a motivator. After thinking about it for days, she opened the piano and gave the keys a tinkle, enjoying the familiar sound. Then she played a well-loved melody. She felt as if she was returning to an old friend and began to play daily.

While she played, a stray terrier stood at the window listening. In spite of her attempts to send the dog away, it returned. Gemma liked the dog and after checking, it seemed to have no home. Eventually she adopted her and called her Amber, due her brown and gold colouring. With music back in its prime place and a dog to keep her company, Gemma's life was fuller and richer, but she had not yet ventured out of the house.

Amber sat at Gemma's feet with her ear cocked as Gemma played. She followed Gemma about the house and slept at the end of her bed at night. She was affectionate and loyal, but an active, young terrier who needed exercise. The dog's insistent nagging to go out, drew Gemma to the front door. Then she stepped onto the grass tentatively and threw an old tennis ball for the dog to chase. When she ventured further, she was delighted that the garden was even lovelier in reality than it seemed through the window. A mass of flowers in bloom and buds she hadn't seen before thrilled her. With Amber yapping and tugging at her clothing, she struggled further.

Roger, who lived across the road from Gemma, heard her playing the piano and was impressed. The start of their friendship began when he knocked on Gemma's door to "compliment the pianist". He was a violinist in the city's symphony orchestra and appreciated her ability. Roger and Gemma had much to share and he became a frequent visitor. With his encouragement, Gemma eventually reached the garden fence. The first time she walked though her front gate onto the pavement outside the house, they drank a toast to her improvement.

Gemma was doing well, but she had a long way to go before she could perform at the concert hall. Pushing herself too hard made her panicky, but she was conquering her fears, and becoming more optimistic.

Gemma and Roger's relationship blossomed. He was caring and supportive, while he gradually encouraged her independence.

Roger had fallen in love with this shy, talented woman and wanted to help her to return to her former strength.

She played the piano every day, but her recovery was not as quick or easy as she had hoped. There were days, when no amount of coaxing would make her feel more positive. Though she was able to collect her post, and venture out of her gate, she had not managed to go much further. To play in the eisteddfod she would have to travel by car.

When Roger mentioned a short drive through the suburb, it seemed impossible. Like all Gemma's progress, each step took time and perseverance. She had two months of preparation left if she was to perform at the concert hall. Once she was able to leave the house and sit in the car for short periods, Roger took her on short drives with Amber at the back of the car. Then he suggested a drive through the city to the concert hall. Though Gemma thought of several excuses, she finally agreed.

Before leaving home, she filled her handbag with things she thought she might need away from home, like chocolate, bottled water and aspirin. Before they set off, she took deep breaths to control her surging fears. As they drove, she glanced at the busy city she had not seen for so long. When they reached the concert hall, Roger turned the car around and headed back home. Gemma sighed with relief.

They drove to the concert hall several times until the ride seemed more natural and comfortable for her. With only a month left before her performance, she hoped to feel more at ease about the next step, leaving the car and entering the hall. At last they went inside the building to explore the large hall. Ten days before the concert, Roger invited Gemma to hear him play violin in a chamber orchestra in one of the smaller rooms of the concert hall. Anticipation of listening to him play brought thoughts of pleasure, but also fears about visiting an unknown place. Once she was seated and listening to Roger, she lost herself in delight.

She left the concert hall feeling slightly more assured that she would manage to give her own performance.

On the night of the concert, Gemma's desire to hide inside the house to avoid the whole situation was powerful, but she fought her fear. Roger decided to take Amber back stage. While Gemma waited for her cue, she stroked Amber's head. When she was called to perform, she looked back at Roger and Amber, and walked out onto the stage towards the piano. She summoned the courage and began to play.

Gemma's exceptionally fine playing spoke to the soul of everyone in the hall. A standing ovation cured her nerves, as she played again and again, causing a rush of emotion that made her flush with joy and her heart pound with excitement rather than anxiety. The critics raved over her performance.

In her elated mood she accepted Roger's proposal of marriage, on condition that they waited until she was more independent. The positive reports about her performance gave her the will to keep on fighting. Instead of ordering online, she set herself the task of walking to the shops. Once she was able to wander around the village, she wanted to visit the city. It took her longer than she thought to achieve her aims, as she had several setbacks of being afraid to leave the house again, but her spells of fear didn't last as long as they had before. With courage and perseverance, she was able to go the city and visit old friends.Roger waited patiently.

Two years after his proposal, they were married. Gemma looked back to those bleak times and realised how far she had progressed with Roger and Amber's help. She continued to play in many concerts and she and Roger lived together happily.

Skeletons in the Cupboard

Steve sat on the beach, too miserable to notice the soft warm sand or the high crested waves. The almost empty beach echoed his aloneness. Like most young people, Steve had experienced moody spells in the past, but the death of his father, followed by a break up with his girlfriend Rana, who fell for someone else, tipped him over the precipice. Rana had been his first love and closest friend. He was accustomed to being with her and the intimacy they shared. She had supported him through his grief and helped him to feel more complete after the loss of his father. She had been there for him too while his mother had her own grief to come to terms with. Knowing that Rana had rejected him, was too painful to bear.

Everything that had been important to him no longer interested him, and his future looked dark. He even had moments when he thought of walking into the sea and drowning, but somehow he had pushed the thoughts away. His mother had tried several times to make an appointment for him to visit a doctor, but Steve refused, as he had heard from friends that medication would be prescribed, and possibly a visit to a counsellor would be suggested. It wasn't for him.

At sunset, a grey haired fisherman gathered his nets to draw in his catch. It was taxing work, and after securing his fish he walked home wearily. He passed a young man sitting alone on the sand. The next day, he noticed that the young man was there again. The fisherman had suffered hurt in the past and recognised the look of despair.

241

Concerned, he approached the young man. 'Hi I'm Craig…I noticed you here alone on the beach yesterday, and then today again,' he said hesitantly. 'I don't want to butt in…I hope you're okay.'

'I'm fine,' the young man replied.

Craig shook his head doubtfully. 'I'm not so sure.'

'Maybe I'm not doing so well…and…I'm Steve.'

Craig sat next to Steve on the sand. Slowly and haltingly, searching for words that he hoped would help, Craig described the struggles and anguish of his youth. 'Phew! I have lots of unhappy memories of my young days. I don't know why, but I called my misery and pain "old bones," he said, smiling wryly. 'I had a huge imagination in those days…still do.' He rubbed his calloused hands together. 'Maybe I got the idea from my mother. She used to say, "all our problems come from family and feelings we aren't supposed to talk about…they're skeletons locked in the cupboard." He stroked his shaggy beard, looked at the sea as if remembering, and then continued talking. 'When I was your age, I imagined all the bones from my past kicking and banging inside me. What a sharp, nasty feeling! They reminded me that I wasn't free of them. Maybe you've got them too and they're making you sad.'

Steve nodded with a slight shudder. 'Yep…I know about those bones. I've got a few stuck in my gut.'

What he's saying is a bit weird, but I understand only too well.

Craig paused, searching again for the right words. 'I'll bet you'd be pleased to get rid of them. Then maybe you'll be able to move on.'

The sand drifted through Steve's fingers. 'Get rid of them…but how…by magic?'

He's a kind man, but it sounds like hocus pocus.

'Tell you what, I'll be at the harbour working on my boat all Sunday morning. Meet me there, and I'll do my best to help you,' Craig said, pointing. 'There she is, I've called her Survivor.'

Nice name for a boat…and it strikes a chord.

Steve shrugged. 'Maybe.'

I've got nothing else to do on Sunday, so maybe I'll give it a go. Not that I expect anything. I doubt he or anyone can help me.

'We'll take her out…then you'll see,' Craig replied with a wave. Steve watched Craig walk away as the golden ball slipped over the horizon.

The following Sunday, Steve found Craig on his boat. Minutes later Craig dropped anchor and they set out. When no land could be seen, he cut the motor. Steve looked at the endless blue of the sky, the calm water and sighed.

'This is a good spot,' Craig said.

As good as any.

Steve looked at him quizzically, wondering what was going to happen.

'You'll get rid of some of those old bones…the stuff bothering you.'

'Let's go for it then,' Steve said.

I'll try anything.

'Right then, sit on the gunnel,' Craig said, pointing to the edge of the boat. 'Close your eyes and take deep breaths of the fresh sea air. Now think of all those hurts lurking inside of you.' He waved his arms to make his point. 'All those old bones rattling, taking up so much space, and messing up your life.' He watched Steve closely. 'Time to get rid of them. Imagine you're taking all your misery, and throwing it into the deep water. The sea's hungry. It gobbles up everything good and bad.'

Slowly Steve's hands went to his chest. Tears flowed down his cheeks as he made slow, rhythmical movements towards the water. He experienced the sensation of a heavy part of him being torn away, as he imagined throwing some of his sadness into the sea. When he opened his eyes he didn't know how long he'd been drifting. Whatever had happened, his despair had eased. He turned towards the fisherman, touched his arm, and mumbled his thanks.

'Good…good. At least this is a start. Some of it has gone. Let the fish worry now, they eat anything,' Craig said with a smile.

While they talked, Craig noticed the sky darkening and the swells rising. 'We'd better head back, there's a storm on its way.'

They were half way back to the harbour, when huge waves began rocking the boat. Steve was still sitting on the gunnel, when a huge wave tossed him into the swirling water. He struggled to keep afloat. Craig threw him a rope, but he turned his head away, as he wrestled with himself. A large part of him wanted to slip down to the sea bed and rest there, but an inner voice told him to take the hard way, and to fight. He seized the rope and Craig hauled him out of the water. Heaving and spluttering, he collapsed at the bottom of the boat, and fell into an exhausted sleep. On waking, he found that the storm had passed and the sky was clear again.

'I'm starving. Anything to eat?' Steve asked.

Craig had brought sandwiches and beer, and they shared it.

They had just finished eating, when Steve pointed. 'Look over there, at the light over the water.'

A faint golden glow had spread across the sea, highlighting the ripples, and a soft arc of light shone in the sky. An eerie stillness hung in the air. Neither of them spoke. As the light faded, Craig started up the engine and steered the boat back to the beach.

Steve smiled for the first time enjoying the breeze.

Gaining Confidence & Independence

Coming To Terms with Blushing

Bruce warmed his hands in front of his camp fire and contemplated the beauty of the night sky. It was the beginning of his two week camping holiday. He enjoyed being alone with the sounds of birds and insects for company. The simplicity of camping with few traditional comforts, and cooking his meals on an open fire appealed to him. There were so many walks through the mountains, the river, and watching animal and bird life, that his days were crammed with interest and activity.

The bush was peaceful away from the pressures that plagued Bruce in the city. He was a short, stocky man with tentative gestures, and an uncertain smile. He was shy with people, especially strangers. If he became embarrassed or challenged, the tips of his ears turned sharp pink, blotches formed on his face and neck that deepened to scarlet, and sweat poured off him. At those embarrassing moments, he wished a hole would open in the floor and devour him. The more he worried about his blushing, the worse it became. At work he avoided other staff members and embarrassing situations as much as possible, and sat at the very back of the office unnoticed. Before he left for his holiday, his manager complimented him on his excellent work, but Bruce found praise extremely embarrassing. His blush was as red as the diary on the manager's desk.

Bruce was a keen naturalist, and delighted in examining unusual plants or insects. One morning while walking, shrubs with unusually bright pink flowers caught his attention. When he bent to sniff the perfume of a flower, he spotted a dragon lizard on a twig. It was brown with a thorny spine on its back that made it almost indistinguishable from its surroundings. He moved quietly to observe it. When they were threatened, dragon lizards were able to change color so as not to be noticed. Their slow movement and sharp spines were an excellent defence. Then, he noticed another dragon lizard. It was green and rocking on a leaf in the afternoon breeze. He admired how lizards adapted to different environments. He smiled wryly, when he thought of his own way of camouflaging himself. He tried to blend in unnoticed at work in fawn and grey clothing, and keeping quiet in the background.

As Bruce continued his walk, he thought of his shyness as a young child, when he had grabbed his mother tightly, and yelled if she talked to strangers. If visitors came to the house, he would bury himself in the blue velvet curtains hoping that he would be forgotten. He remembered blushing for the first time in junior school when the teacher asked him a question, and then rushing out of the class room humiliated. He thought of the misery of the teasing he had suffered on account of blushing. At university things didn't improve. Mixing with other students made him edgy. In spite of his good grades, he dropped out of university before completing his studies.

By the end of his first week away, Bruce had eaten almost all the tinned and packaged food he had brought with him, but he wasn't concerned. As in previous years, he looked to the bush for food. At the stream, only a short walk away, masses of pink and white waterlilies floated on the surface. They were his first choice. Their stems and roots made a tasty stew. As he picked the waterlilies he must've frightened the cockatoos in the bushes. Their crests turned red and erect in response to the threat of a stranger. He understood their reaction, and tried to move about slowly and quietly.

The following day, he set out to catch fish in the river. He relaxed, enjoying the view of the river and mountain, and ate the lunch he'd brought along with him under a tree. By late afternoon, the sky was streaked with rose and violet. Flocks of birds gathered in the trees waiting for their insect catch. Before leaving with his bag of fish, he took a swig of brandy from his flask, and marveled at the kaleidoscope of colour and shadow. Sighing with pleasure, he sniffed the air, expecting to smell the twilight scent of wild flowers, but instead his sensitive nose detected smoke.

A thin plume of smoke rose from a group of caravans parked on a nearby farm. He dropped his fish, and ran in the direction of the smoke. A bale of hay had caught alight. Flames were rising, and had jumped the fence close to the caravans. As no one was about, Bruce assumed that they were cooking their evening meal and hadn't noticed the fire. He raced between the caravans loudly shouting "fire". There were shrieks as the campers ran out of their caravans. Some of the older people needed help. He ripped at a rope with his pocket knife to free a woman whose leg was caught. He grabbed a terrified child screaming, wrapped her in his jacket, and took her out in his arms. Once everyone was safe, he helped to put out the fire. Then he slipped away. Rescuing people in an emergency situation was something he had not imagined himself doing.

The next morning, water was boiling on the fire for his breakfast, when a group of people from the caravan camp came to thank him. He shared his meal with them, and they all sat talking while they ate. He now had a group of new friends who wanted to show him the best fishing spots and places to view small game. Bruce spent the last few days of his holiday walking and examining the plants and wild life with his friends. He couldn't have imagined a more enjoyable holiday.

He ate his last meal as the early sun peeped through the night sky. As he packed his four wheel drive, he was reluctant to leave the freedom of the open spaces, but more optimistic than he had been for a long while. He had seen himself at his best, and it had given him a burst of new confidence.

When he returned to work, he asked to be moved into the body of the office. Without challenges, he knew that he would never get over his problem. He struggled to communicate with others in the office at first. Talking to women made him self-conscious, and he still blushed occasionally. Women found his pink cheeks endearing, and he made a few female friends. He knew he was overcoming his problem when he bought his first blue striped shirt, and joined his work mates for a beer after work.

Margaret Goes On Strike

Margaret watched the thick line of ants filing across the window ledge, over the shutter and down the wall, absorbed in their movements, as they scurried behind each other.

That's me, just one of many racing to keep going.

It would be another day at work, fitting in her household chores, and insufficient time to spend with her children. It worried her that when her children came home from school in the afternoon she wasn't there to give them the attention they needed. That the house didn't meet her usual high standard of neatness and cleanliness bothered her too. So many things had become responsibilities and obligations to others that she fulfilled without question. Over weekends, she helped her husband with his accounts. Twice a week after work, she squeezed in a visit to her father in hospital. The demands on her had taken their toll, and at the end of the day she was so tired that she barely managed to cook the evening meal. Though she fell into bed exhausted each night, she slept poorly and felt tired when she woke.

Her work had been enjoyable, and she had been an efficient personal assistant, until a new computer system was introduced. Not only were records thrown into chaos, but she was forced to learn a totally different approach. Learning was slow and tedious. For the first time, she dreaded work each day. Nothing had the order she once knew, and all her efforts seemed for nothing.

One Friday, she decided to take a proper lunch break. She usually grabbed a sandwich and coffee and worked through lunch, but this time she wanted to shake off a gloominess that was weighing her down. It was a warm day, and the streets were throbbing with shoppers. She passed elegant shops, but didn't stop to look in their windows as she once had.

At a sidewalk café, she sat in the sunshine under a striped awning. As she spooned up the froth of her cappuccino, she heard sounds of marching and loud hailers a few blocks away. She gulped down her coffee, and left the café to follow the sounds. Members of the Garment Workers Union were on strike, and a mob of women protesters were stomping and yelling their demands.

As a young woman, her mother had worked as a machinist in a factory. She told Margaret about the strain of making every seam straight in the fastest possible time, and working long hours. Margaret nodded to herself. She knew how it felt to be undervalued, both at home and in her job. As she watched the enthusiastic crowd, she felt the throb of their excitement. In minutes, she was caught up in the mood of the march. Without thinking, she joined in shouting with them, *Slave labour. Less time more money.* She rarely shouted, and didn't display her feelings in public, but this was different.

They surged past a tall building displaying a clock face. It was 2.10 p.m. , time to return to the office, but she continued to keep pace with the others. Finally the line of strikers thinned.

She clenched her fist.

I've had enough of the new computer programme, and allowing myself to be used by my family. Its time I did something about it... stood up for myself, showed them how I feel.

She made an instant decision. *I'm going on strike too.*

Margaret left work early. In the train home, waves of weariness swept over her and tears of resentment flowed down her cheeks, as she sank into the seat. She walked slowly from the station to her house. Once home, she placed her handbag on the hall table, and went straight to the bedroom. Her overriding thought was of slipping into bed. She closed her eyes and thought about her husband Dennis, who expected her to do all the housework and cooking as well as her work. Her two lazy teenage sons were usually sprawled out in front of the television nibbling snack food. Their vague offers to help in the house had been given such a long time ago that she had forgotten.

She stretched and yawned.

It's time for them to take over. I'm not doing another thing. She smiled. Down go my household tools – the iron, saucepan, vacuum, everything that cleans, cooks or chugs.

In a dream sleep, her mother was standing before her, large and overbearing. Margaret was younger and small. "Lying around idle again. There's work to be done in the house, my girl. Get up!"

In the dream, she meekly followed her mother's instructions.

"Come with me!" her mother said, as she walked around the house running her finger along glass tops and furniture. "This hasn't been dusted for days." Her mother straightened a few paintings and reorganised the cushions on the sofa, before walking towards the door. "I'll leave you to it, then."

Margaret woke seething with resentment.

Why can't she leave me alone now that she's dead?

When Dennis came home from work to find her in bed, he was stunned. He took one look at her pale face, and urged her to make an appointment to see her doctor.

The doctor spoke kindly to her about looking after herself in the future. He told her that the stresses of working plus caring for her home and her family could make her seriously ill if she didn't rest.

'Definitely, two weeks off work and total rest…then we'll decide,' he said. 'I'd like to see you before you even consider going back to work.'

She returned to bed. That night, Dennis sat on the edge of the bed struggling to find words to tell her how worried he was, and how much he cared for her. Later, he brought her tea and roughly cut sandwiches. Between tears, she told him how tired she was, and that for a while she couldn't face looking after him, and the boys or the house. He admitted that he had no idea where to start, but he wanted her to rest. He promised that he and the boys would do their best to manage.

That day and the next, she lay in bed feeling drained, yet uncomfortable about relaxing. Lying in bed was foreign to her. She believed that women who gave in to minor illnesses were weak. Her mother visited her several times in dreams, always reprimanding her. Each time, she was filled with a mixture of guilt and resentment.

She slept more than she could remember. Even if she wanted to clean and cook her energy had deserted her. She felt guilty about not visiting her father in hospital too, and phoned instead.

Dennis and the boys applied themselves to most of the household chores. They mastered the dishwasher and vacuum cleaner, but struggled at first with sorting clothes for the washing machine. Dennis bought take-away food for two nights, then he longed for a solid meal. At the supermarket he bought frozen vegetables, chips and three huge slices of steak. She was astounded when he turned out a tasty meal. Dennis also visited his father-in-law in hospital. Though it pleased her to see her men as they went about their chores, she feared that their dedication wouldn't last.

When she saw the doctor again, he wasn't satisfied with her progress. He insisted on at least another two weeks at home. Gradually she left her bed, watched a little television, and read a book. The thought of returning to work made her apprehensive.

Around that time, Margaret had another dream about her mother. This time her mother's comments no longer upset her.

'So what have you been doing all this time?'

'Resting Mother. It's what the doctor said I need to do.'

'Humph', was the reply as her mother wandered round the house looking in corners and testing for dust. 'Clean enough, but not sparkling.'

'It's time you left me to run my house,' Margaret snapped. Miffed, her mother turned and walked off.

The dream amused Margaret. She pictured her mother with a duster in one hand, a cleaning cloth in the other, as she wiped surfaces with antiseptic, or cleaned under furniture searching for hidden dirt. The beds had to be made before she left in the morning, and at least one load of washing had to be done. Her mother hardly ever sat down, and if she did it, it wasn't for long.

It was the first time Margaret had laughed, or even smiled for weeks. Stronger and more optimistic, she began to enjoy her late sleeps, reading and occasional walks.

Dennis called a family meeting. There were hugs all round and expressions of pleasure about Margaret's improved health. Everyone agreed that before she considered returning to work, a roster ought to be drawn up to share the responsibilities of managing the house. Dennis and her sons insisted on taking on most of the home management between them, and left Margaret the remainder. The roster was to be reviewed as she grew stronger. She was proud that Dennis was turning into an efficient housekeeper, and her sons were taking an active part in running their home.

That night, she had her last dream about her mother. They were in the sitting room having tea. Her mother was white haired, small and frail, as she had been before she died. They chatted pleasantly, and then kissed each other goodbye. Margaret woke feeling relieved, but sad at seeing her mother so fragile.

When Margaret saw the doctor again, they both agreed that she could return to work, but for mornings only. Her boss and the office staff welcomed her. During her month away she had been missed, and two replacements were required to do her job. Her boss happily agreed to her working mornings only, and employed one of the women who had replaced her while she was away. Even the shorter working hours tired her. Though she was home in time for a late lunch, most afternoons she needed to rest. Weeks later, she managed her few chores after work.

Work became easier, but Margaret didn't increase her hours. She wanted more time to herself, and to feel less pressured. Her boss was satisfied with their arrangement. The new computer system seemed less daunting and she mastered it in her own time.

With her family helping out, and less work pressure, her sense of humour and capacity to enjoy life returned. A plus was Dennis' new hobby, cooking. He had a natural flair. She couldn't believe her luck. Four times a week, he cooked the evening meal. Soon she took over more household tasks, but not all of them. A good deal had been negotiated, and she often wondered if the members of the Garment Workers Union had done as well with their strike.

The Suit

There was once a very old man with leathery, wrinkled skin, but a sharp memory. In spite of the aches and pains of age, he was happy. Storytelling came to him naturally, and he captivated his audiences with tales of wars, famines, great struggles and his own achievements. The story he enjoyed telling most often was about his battle to overcome painful memories of his past.

'On my twenty-first birthday, my parents gave me a gift of a navy, pin-striped suit. It was made of fine wool, and designed by the best tailors, but I disliked it from the moment I opened the box. When I tried it on it fitted perfectly, but it was far too formal. The stripes made me feel locked in. It wasn't my style. I preferred casual clothing, and put it at the back of my cupboard, but I didn't forget about it.

Let's leave the suit in the cupboard, while I tell you a bit about myself. I had a wonderful childhood, playing games after school, and riding my bike with my mates. My parents weren't affectionate, but they cared for me well enough. I never went hungry.

Shortly after I turned nine, my life changed. What happened to me at nine, you may ask. Well, my father was a sailor, and one night when he was away at sea, my uncle came to stay, as he often did. I couldn't sleep that night, and on the way to the kitchen for some milk I passed my mother's bedroom. There I saw my mother and uncle in bed. I don't need to go into details, because you'll know the noises I heard, and what I saw when I peeped through the keyhole. None of it was pretty to my young eyes. I was shocked, repulsed and angry all at once. I hated my uncle, and was ashamed and disappointed in my mother.

After that night, I could barely look at my uncle, and though I still loved my mother, I no longer respected her. I kept thinking of my father, working on a ship far from home unaware of what was happening. It upset me deeply, and in many ways changed me. From being a fun-loving boy with lots of friends, I turned into a withdrawn, sad one. I trusted no one. My school results plummeted, and I was dumped from the football team.

Later, when I was working, I didn't date much. Over weekends I hardly went to football or the movies.

A few months after my twenty-first birthday, an older man joined our company. He sat next to me, and talked a lot about his life, and his recollections of the war. I didn't say much, just listened. He had been to one of those head doctors who helped him to overcome his nightmares. The doc told him to let his memories of the war into his dreams...in little bits at a time. All I know is that he got rid of most of the dark stuff worrying him.

I thought about him, and reckoned that it was time for me to change too, but I had no idea where to start. Perhaps changes in me began when I went to my sister's wedding. The navy suit came out of the cupboard. It fitted me perfectly. With a pink carnation and a tie it suited the occasion. After the wedding, I began to have the strangest dreams. It's hard to believe I know, but I dreamt about that navy suit often. My early dreams about the suit are still clear. I took it out of the cupboard, shook the dust from it, hung it up to air, and put it back again.

Then my dreams changed. I saw a reenactment of my mother and uncle in bed, caught in the suit's pockets. I tried to tear off the pockets, but couldn't. I woke in a sweat, my heart thumping. After that dream I couldn't think about putting my hand in a pocket without flinching.

About a year later, I was promoted at work and invited to the company's Christmas dinner. I had only one good suit, the navy striped one. The most peculiar thing happened when I tried the suit on the night before the dinner. I hadn't put on any weight, but the suit felt tight and uncomfortable. The sleeves and legs seemed short. It was probably my imagination, and imagination can do the weirdest things. Though there was nothing wrong with the suit, I knew I couldn't wear it. Luckily, I was able to hire a suit in time for the occasion.

My dreams about the suit continued, but now little tears appeared along the seams.

I had gained confidence in my job by then, and my dreams about the suit changed again. I dreamed that I was trying to rub the pin stripes out of the material. It was a huge job, but each night I erased a few more stripes. It must have taken ages, but when they were all gone, in my dreams, that is, I woke feeling good.

I began to enjoy life. I dated a woman from work, but our relationship fizzled out. It was my fault. Somehow I couldn't allow myself to trust her. After that I took a long break from women.

Did I tell you about my drinking? It began slowly with a few beers after work or with my meal. When I had to nip out to the hotel for a drink every lunch time, I knew I was in trouble. It became expensive, but I didn't spend on anything else, so I could afford my habit. Most of the males in my family were drunks, but that didn't excuse it. I knew I had to give up drinking. I didn't have an option.

The withdrawal period was tough, with the shakes, being irritable and jumpy. I couldn't go back to work for weeks. For no reason I'd get resentful or very sad, and want to cry. Then I'd battle for hours to calm down. It felt as if a painful oozing wound inside me hadn't healed yet.

My suit dreams at the time were bizarre. The navy material pulled in all directions and wound itself into knots. White heat escaped from the suit until the seams burst. My dreams mirrored my feelings.

With help, I managed to stay off the booze, but couldn't touch as much as a drop in case I started drinking again. I've slipped back a few times, but these days I don't go near the stuff. After that, my life went along quietly enough for a time, and I became aware of small pleasures - a long, hot shower, a full moon and stars, walking in the rain and listening to music. I was like a kid again. The suit dreams stopped for a while.

It must've been around that time, that I worked up the courage to visit my uncle. He was old by then, but I told the bastard what I thought of him. Do you know, he didn't remember sleeping with his sister-in-law all those years ago. It was amazing how facing him lifted an enormous burden from me. The painful sting had gone from my memory.

I expect you want to know what happened to the real suit. Well, other than being old fashioned, it stayed the same, stripes and all. I was moving ahead. After the meeting with my uncle, I went through a growth spurt. I was in my forties, so it was about time it happened. I started dating again and met my wife-to-be, Nancy. I loved her and after two years I learned to trust her. Once we were married we made friends with other couples and our life together was happy.

Every now and again, I had a suit dream. I'd turn out the pockets, throw away the contents, and clean the bits of lint that had collected in the trouser turn-ups. The dreams no longer bothered me. I smiled to myself when I woke from them. I was doing a bit of inner cleaning, that's all.

My last and most dramatic suit dream was in my late fifties, and I remember it clearly. The suit's front buttons glowed, fell off and then melted. I was at peace after that.

About eight years ago, I pulled the suit out of my cupboard. Though it was old fashioned, it was still in good condition. I'd hung on to it for far too long. I gave it to the Salvation Army and was pleased to get rid of it.

After telling his story the old man was tired. Those listening asked questions about the suit, but he smiled and didn't answer.

Carole and Mr. Woody

The sun oozed through early clouds, blossoms were on show, and every green thing in the garden was sprouting. Carole sat on the grass wiping away a few tears. Thank goodness the summer holidays had started with a break from university. At least she'd have a rest from facing the bullies. At twenty-one she felt embarrassed telling anyone what was happening to her. She hid it from her family, and very few of her friends knew that she was being bullied.

She was in her final year of a teaching course, and a group of mean girls were spoiling it for her. She was different to most of the other young women in her group. Dressing in the latest fashion, and using make up wasn't important to her. To most of the others, her interest in debating, ecology and world events appeared strange. When at first, a few of the women made snide remarks about her hairstyle or dress sense, she brushed them off. But that wasn't the end of it. They ignored her, turned their backs on her, or bumped into her on purpose to make her drop her books. It was the sort of thing children did. She couldn't believe that they were behaving in that way.

Later, Carole was having a cup of coffee on the patio, staring aimlessly at the sky, when she saw it. A blob circling, and then like a dive bomber it made its landing a few metres from her. It was a duck. They stared at each other. She held her ground uncertainly. But it didn't squawk or show signs of attack. All she heard was a steady 'pluck, pluck'. It waddled, turning itself around several times so that she could appreciate its features. It had white feathers, mottled with brown, a dark head and beak, masked eyes and teal on its side. A beauty! She guessed the duck was a male, as they were usually the better looking birds.

She dashed into the kitchen for stale bread she kept for the many birds that visited. After wetting the bread, she dropped it on the grass and waited. Meanwhile, the duck was luxuriating in the rock pool at the top of the garden. Only after he'd ruffled his feathers, preened himself and scanned the garden, did he nibble the bread. After his meal, the duck waddled nonchalantly onto a grassy strip and took off.

Carole didn't expect to see the duck again, but he flew in each day during her break from studies. She looked forward to his visits and gave him the name of Mr. Woody. He followed the same pattern. After eating his ration of bread, he paddled in the pool. The duck was almost tame by then. Some days he followed her inside, but ignored her on others.

'You're a strange one Mr. Woody. You do exactly as you like,' she said, laughing and throwing the duck another piece of bread.

Two days before university resumed, his visits stopped. Carole scoured the skies but no blob was visible. She wondered about the duck's arrival the day holidays began, and its disappearance shortly before she was due to go back to her studies.

With the break almost over, she began to worry about the bullies.

I've enjoyed the freedom from them. But they probably haven't grown up during the break.

By now Carole knew her inner voice well. It usually warned her about people who were nasty, or if she had done the wrong thing. This time her inner voice told her that there was something to learn from Mr. Woody's visit.

Spread your wings, the voice niggled. And don't worry about the others. Keep being an individual and don't pander to the bullies.

Carole returned to university with Mr. Woody in mind. She walked past the bullies with her head held high imagining she was ruffling her feathers, and ignored them. Water off a duck's back, she told herself, laughing at the cliché. She didn't even look back to see if they reacted. The bullies must've read her message of new confidence and didn't approach her again. Carole forgot about them.

She passed her final exam with excellent grades and decided to study further. By the following summer she was enjoying university life. One afternoon when she was home earlier than usual, the duck visited. It followed her into the kitchen and waited for bread.

Twins

Sixteen-year-old Felicity and Deirdre were twins who were not identical in looks or temperament. They lived with their parents on a farm with a magnificent view of the countryside. Deirdre was slim and serious with dark hair that hung loosely over her shoulders, while Felicity was easy going and fun loving, and wore her curly blonde hair short. In spite of their differences, the twins had a deep connection and each knew how the other thought and felt.

They did most things together and lived contentedly until late one afternoon a ferocious storm struck the farm. As wild lightening flashed followed by bellowing thunder, they hid under the bed they shared. They held each other in terror, as beams snapped, walls buckled, and wild winds lifted the ceiling. After the storm, the girls were not hurt, but their home was in ruins. Frantically, they searched for their parents. They found them in the barn – dead, struck by lightning, together with dead goats and sheep. The twins clung to each other and wept. There was no time for mourning. They did not seek out a priest, but buried their parents on the hillside the following day, and placed wild flowers and a boulder on each of the graves to mark the spot. Their neighbours helped them to bury many of their dead animals.

Now that their parents were dead, they cared for each other. Fortunately, the insurance company paid them enough to build a new house. While builders from the town constructed their house, they stayed in a shelter they made from the wood and bricks that littered the hillside after the storm. The new house was designed to be small and functional, and able to withstand further attacks by nature. While they waited for their house, the girls worked tirelessly, caring for the surviving animals, as well as removing debris and trees the storm had ripped from the ground.

Once they moved into their new home they rested, and for the first time they were able to reflect on the tragedy of their parent's death. The twins believed that they had been saved for a reason, but exactly what the reason was, became a subject of many late night discussions.

After settling in, they met their neighbours and formed some close friendships. Gradually they took part in country life, attending fairs, concerts and dinners. Each sister had boyfriends, but there was no place for husbands. They managed the farm together. Though they were opposites, they maintained a balance in both the farm and in their lives.

Deirdre, the more practical twin was concerned about weather forecasts, the cost of fodder and the quality of the soil. Felicity, the more fun loving and inventive sister was inspired by a string of new ideas for developing the farm. She wanted to plant exotic flowers in a hot house, keep llamas, and create a restaurant for tourists. Deirdre listened carefully to her sister's suggestions, and sifted out only the most practical of her many ideas.

Deirdre discouraged both the llamas and restaurant suggestions, but encouraged Felicity to build a large hothouse and grow the flowers in demand. When the flowers sold well at the market, they built a second and larger hothouse. The farm flourished. Deirdre attended to the administration and the sales of their animals, flowers and crops, while Felicity supervised the day to day farming, often working side by side with the farmhands.

'We're a great balance for each other, and together we've created a thriving business,' Felicity said one day as they were walking through their land.

'Very true,' Deirdre replied solemnly.

The twins remained happy and healthy until they reached the age of fifty-five, when aches and pains surfaced. When they discussed their physical changes, they realised that they could both lose some weight. They began to eat more simply and lived together contentedly until they were sixty-four. While Deirdre was climbing a ladder to search for documents, she lost her balance, fell, and hit her head. She was airlifted to hospital, but died three days later.

Felicity was distraught. She had not been alone for more than two days, and ached for her twin as intensely as if one of her limbs had been sawn off. Her emotions were so disturbed, that she felt that the destructive storm they had survived in their youth had returned.

Gradually time began to heal the wound of Felicity's loss. Everything the twins had taught each other remained with her, and she continued to run the farm. The balance they had achieved was now part of her, and she was grateful. After a year of solitude, Felicity grew tired of being alone, and accepted dinner invitations in the district. It was at one of these dinners that she met Spence. They had a brief courtship and married in the spring, exactly three years after Deirdre's death. Though Felicity and Spence loved each other, Deirdre's spirit continued to live within her, sharing experiences and guiding her until her death twenty years later.

Connections with the Past

The Phone Call

Paul checked his watch. Another morning shift at the alcohol rehabilitation centre was over. He left through the side door and pulled his woolen cap down over his balding head to avoid the sharp wind. He had worked at the centre as a volunteer for twenty-one years, four days a week. During the early stages of alcohol withdrawal, the patients needed intense, caring nursing to get then through the shakiness, confusion, fast heart rate and fever that marked the feared DT's. Later, Paul provided the emotional support they needed, stilling their fears and bringing them back to focus on what was really important, their recovery, and then abstinence. Over the years he had slipped into the role of a lay counsellor.

He took the long route home, as he did most days, avoiding the park where children played, often unaccompanied by adults. Avoiding the park was one of the ways he disciplined himself. Then he stopped at the church where he found comfort in prayer, and in following the rituals that had been part of his life. The church was empty. All he heard was his own breathing.

After his prayers, he sat for a while thinking of his childhood, and of the four generations of clergy in his family. He smiled, remembering his sweet soprano voice at seven, and singing at the church choir concerts when the audience clapped loudly. Then he was holding his grandfather's hand in church, while his father spoke at the pulpit. He recalled the community picnics at the beach with sandwiches, cream donuts, muffins with blueberries, and fizzy lemonade. The memory of the time he was dumped in the sea by a bunch of girls who thought he'd become too full of himself made him smile again.

Then his mind slipped back further to the Easter when the family was invited to Great Aunt Edith and Uncle Edgar's farm. He and the other children had played at the creek at the sharp end of their property, while the adults talked and drank red wine. His family slept over at the farm that night, and a bed was made up for him in a small back room.

As he slept, a sudden heaviness had awakened him. It was his father, smelling strongly of alcohol. At first, the stroking on his naked skin had been pleasurable, but when fingers became intrusive touching and probing private places, he struggled unsuccessfully to wriggle away. There were many other dark memories of his father's visits, but as he grew older and stronger he defended himself, and pushed his father away.

Though he didn't speak to his father again, he fulfilled his obligations and studied for the priesthood. There were many pleasing memories during the period of intense spirituality of his studies. He recalled working for his first congregation, being well liked and effective. Within a few years he had built up a large church choir as well. It was his happiest time.

Less pleasurable were his recollections of choir practice when he had first felt aberrant urges, overwhelming diabolical thoughts and feelings about the choirboys. He saw himself playing out his own past. How naïve he had been not to predict that some of the boys would tell their parents about the touches, pats and gentle squeezes. There had been only one brief meeting with the bishop, his most painful memory. His life as a priest ended. He was being transferred to the city's Diocese Library, and he tried to start again in a distant part of the city.

It was late afternoon when Paul left the church. Still deep in thought, he was unaware of the swaying trees, or the sting of the wind. All he noticed was his pounding guilt.

Once home, he withdrew into safety. He followed his routine at home of eating alone, having one glass of wine with his meal, and another after. Then he read or listened to relaxing music.

When a letter arrived inviting him to the centre's twentieth birthday celebration, he was delighted. A number of volunteers were to be honoured guests, and he was one of them. He thought about the dinner for days beforehand, wondering who would be there. When at last the evening arrived, he was shown to a seat at a front table. After dinner the speeches began. Paul and several other loyal volunteers were thanked and given silver badges. When he pinned his badge onto his coat, a few tears wet his face. Would he ever do enough to compensate for his transgressions?

One evening, while he was enjoying his second glass of wine, the jarring sound of the telephone startled him. He hardly ever received phone calls.

'I'd like to speak to Mr. Horton please,' the caller said.

'Who's calling?'

'Evan King here.'

'How can I help you?'

'I'm looking for Paul Horton…priest and choirmaster many years ago?'

There was a brief silence before Paul replied. 'A choirmaster? You have the wrong number.'

Evan probed. 'Are you certain you didn't lead the choir back in the late fifties or sixties?'

Paul began to feel clammy. 'No…no! I'm a volunteer at a rehabilitation centre. Before that I worked at a library.'

'Well, sorry to have disturbed you.' Evan said.

'That's okay,' Paul said in his kindest voice.

Paul replaced the phone and collapsed into the nearby armchair. If I'm lucky he won't phone again, he thought.

As summer and autumn passed, Paul forgot about the phone call. On a rainy cold winter's night the phone rang. It was Evan King. Once again Paul insisted he had worked as a librarian before retiring.

'I've been doing some research . . . and it points to you. I'd like to sort it out,' Evan said, speaking loudly.

'Horton isn't an unusual a name, you know. There are lots of us. There must be some mistake,' Paul insisted.

'Maybe…but not in Melbourne. I've already phoned all the P. Hortons.' Evan sounded agitated.

'Why are you looking for this person, anyway?' Paul tried to sound concerned.

'To put things straight…this bastard priest, cum choir master abused me when I was a child, and it still preys on my mind,' Evan said, his voice heavy with emotion.

Paul tried to sound shocked. 'Abused you! Oh my goodness, how absolutely awful. I'm so sorry to learn that. You must've been through a lot.'

Evan struggled to speak. 'I can't tell you how much. I think about it most days and it keeps me awake at night. It never leaves me.'

'Now I can understand why you're so desperate to find this man. Who can blame you after such a terrible experience.' Paul hoped he sounded genuine.

'I couldn't be more desperate. He has to pay for what he's done to me, and probably to others too.' There was pain in Evan's voice.

Paul tried to calm himself as he asked. 'Have you been to the police about this?'

'They told me they can't prosecute someone who doesn't exist. So I need to find out where the bastard lives.'

Paul took a deep breath before speaking again. 'I guess that's logical…he might be dead by now for all you know…still, it's hard to take.'

'You have no idea.'

Paul thought of the counselling skills he used at the centre, and tried again. 'It's not good for you to be so distressed, and to carry all these dreadful memories around inside you, Evan. They can fester. Maybe you'd feel better if you unburdened yourself. Have you thought of talking to someone about it?'

'No, not really,' Even said.

'We men feel we have to be strong, you know and … we don't like to admit to feeling hurt or distressed,' Paul said, trying harder to be empathic.

'That's quite true. I haven't spoken about it to anyone. You're the first.' Evan replied.

'Well, thank you for sharing your pain with me,' Paul said in his most gentle and caring voice. I know it's not my place to suggest it, but perhaps you should consider talking to a counsellor. They're trained to help us overcome things like this.'

'Yes, I have to get over it.' Evan's voice was laden with emotion.

'I'm sure you will…I can hear it in your voice.'

There was silence until Evan spoke again. 'You know, it's been really good talking to you tonight. It must've been luck that I phoned, because I feel better already. I'll see someone about it soon.'

Paul tried to find the right words. 'Why suffer Evan when you can get some help. We live in modern times now, and no one judges a person who goes to a counsellor.'

'Well thanks again Mr. Horton. You've been very kind to help me… and given me something to think about.'

Paul sighed with relief, hoping he'd sent Evan on a different track. 'It's a pleasure Evan…a real pleasure. Now you be sure to take good care of yourself.'

'Yes, thank you. I'll keep hunting for that choirmaster, but get some help too. Goodnight.'

Paul sighed with relief, stretched for the wine bottle, and poured a full glass. A day later, he had a peephole in his door and a deadlock installed. He changed his phone number too, and made certain it was silent. In spite of constant requests, he stopped working at the rehabilitation centre. A visit to the church was too risky, he thought, and he didn't return. Apart from an occasional quick walk on the beach and a visit to the small supermarket two blocks away he stayed at home, a prisoner.

Nadja and her Greyhound

'This is Jewel,' Nadja told her friend Edna as she stroked the sleeping Greyhound's head. The two friends first met at a dog rescue centre, where they were volunteers.

'He's an amber beauty,' Edna said, looking at the large dog with his head perched on Nadja's feet. 'Jewel is a lovely name.'

'I called him Jewel, because he's been a jewel to me. He changed my life in so many ways,' Nadja said, as she stroked the dog again. 'He came into the rescue centre on a cold day, shivering, and looking hungry. I asked the staff about him. They told me that he was about three years old and that he'd been a racing dog. It seems that his owners didn't want him. He was found wandering the street without any identification.'

'Poor thing! Some owners can be cruel to racing dogs if they aren't fast enough or cost a lot to feed.' Edna said.

Nadja added. 'I was concerned about him and went to his cage to see what I could do for him. He had finished a huge meal and was lying on his mat. I thought he was beautiful with that elegant head of his, glowing eyes and elongated body. But he'd lost so much weight that I could see his bones.'

'So sad,' Edna said shaking her head.

'I spoke to him softly. His ears pricked up and his tail wagged ever so slightly. I continued talking and was surprised that he came up to the wire of the cage, and pushed his nose through to touch my hand. I care about all the dogs and bring them treats, but there was something different about this dog. I felt a connection with him.'

Edna nodded.

'Every day I visited him and took him for walks, even though the staff feared he would pull away from me and run off. He walked next to me and didn't even tug the lead. I waited for his owners to claim him, but when they didn't I decided to adopt him. I knew he would need a lot of care and exercise, but I wanted him, and had made up my mind to have him. When I took him home, he was nervous at first, but he's happy and settled now, and that's the main thing.'

'It seems like you did the right thing by following your heart and adopting Jewel,' Edna said.

Nadja thought of the first time she had seen him run. She had taken him for long walks, but hadn't allowed him to run until he had settled in his new home. For his first run, she chose a nearby sports oval with a sandy path where they had walked several times. When she took off his lead, he looked at her and waited. When she said loudly "go…run" he took off at an athletic sprint, disappeared and then was back next to her.

Edna looked puzzled. 'He's a beautiful dog, but why did you say he changed your life?' she asked.

'It's a long story…and if you want to hear it, I'd better make a cup of tea,' Nadja said, looking sad for the first time.

'I could do with a cup, and then please tell me your story.'

Nadja sipped her tea as she talked. 'I was born in Bosnia thirty-six years ago. My sister Zahida and I are the only ones in our family who survived the civil war in our country. I was twelve years old when we arrived in Australia in 1994.

'So sorry you lost your family members. I don't know much about the war,' Edna said.

'Well, in 1992, after all the conflict, the government of Bosnia-Herzegovina declared independence from Yugoslavia, and all hell broke out. The Bosnian Serb forces, backed by the Serb-controlled Yugoslav army attacked Muslims like us, and the Croatians. They called it "ethnic cleansing"…but actually it was a terrible act of genocide.'

'Oh, how dreadful! You must've had a terrible time.' Edna looked shocked.

'Memories of the war don't leave me. It's worst if something triggers a memory. Then it's happening again…the Serbian military storming into our village, burning our houses, killing our men, and raping our women. I cry when I think of how my father and two brothers were killed in the hills around Srebrenica.'

Nadja sighed before continuing. 'One of my worst recollections is when the army forced my mother, my sister Zahida, little Maida aged two, and me, into a sport stadium packed with many other women. It was hot and dirty, and there was no food or water. Maida, developed a dreadful fever and was dead within hours. We couldn't even bury her. After three days, the Serbian troops drove all of us in trucks to a huge forest. With so many bodies crammed together in the trucks for three hours over rough terrain, my mother fainted. She died a week later of a fever. Only Zahida and me were left, and kind people helped us through the forest. We ate rats cooked over a fire and roots until we made it to the United Nations safe zone. After that we were taken to hospital, then a refugee camp, but I hardly remember that.'

Edna asked, 'So how did you come to Sydney?'

'We were accepted as refugees to Australia. Kind Muslims agreed to be our foster parents, and they eventually adopted us. We learned English and went to school here. The adjustment was hard, but we had help and managed. I was too confused to be interested in making friends, or later, any relationships. But, Zahida has many friends, she's married and has two children. I was lucky to win a scholarship to study at university. I became a teacher and enjoyed my work. But I was still nervous, on the lookout for danger and didn't respond well to the children. They called me "Cold Fish." But just as well things have changed since Jewel came into my life.'

'I'm so sorry this happened to you Nadja, but thank goodness you found Jewel,' Edna said, as she took her friend's hand.

Jewel must've heard his name and woke slowly wagging his tail when he saw the two women.

'He's a gentle dog and so sensitive to my moods. He cuddles up when I'm sad and I feel better. He's funny too. Imagine this big dog tying to sit on my lap like a puppy.'

Edna laughed.

'Since I've had him, I'm not so afraid. He's protective and I trust him to listen for me. I have bad dreams less often now,' Nadja said.

Edna nodded. 'That's wonderful! My dogs are my protectors too, and so loyal.'

'After school and weekends he gets me out of the house. I've made new friends in the park when I take him for a run. The most important change is that through his loving I've learned to feel again. I was dead inside after the war, but my love for Jewel changed me. There are people like you Edna, who I can open up to now. The children at school seem to like me more...and I even have a boyfriend,' Nadja said with a laugh.

Edna gave Nadja a hug. 'It seems like you have given each other a new chance...a new life. Jewel had no future in the dog refuge, and you were struggling. Now things have changed for you both and that's wonderful. I think we need something stronger than a cup of tea for a toast!'

The Fruits of the Past

It was Sunday night in Jerusalem. A hit song blared from the packed vegetarian bistro while aromas of hummus, cumin, cinnamon, sugar, and coconut vied with onions, lemon, and pomegranate. Yoni and Dan, in their early twenties, owned the bistro. Both their parents were working when they were growing up and as children they began cooking for their families. Later, they enjoyed experimenting with recipes, which stood them in good stead in the bistro. Their healthy vegetarian dishes made with legumes, beans, and chickpeas in a variety of flavoursome dishes drew locals and tourists alike.

One busy night, oil spilled onto the bistro floor, but in the small kitchen no one noticed it. Yoni was creating one of his special appetisers, when he slipped on the oil slick, and fell on the concrete floor. The severe pain in his right hand and arm told him that he had broken his wrist. An x-ray confirmed his fears. His right wrist was broken in two places, which meant he had a cast from his fingers to his forearm. The worst part was that he was unable to work.

At first, he tried to help at the bistro, but his presence and occasional interference, though well-meant, made the staff edgy. After a long conversation with Dan, he decided to visit his home, Arad, for the six weeks while his arm was in plaster.

He and his mother had been close and no matter how busy he was, he had made time to talk to her daily on the phone and he went to see her regularly. When she died, two years earlier, he threw himself into work to block his grief. The last time he went to Arad was for his mother's funeral, but he had left soon after.

Though Arad was only a few hours drive from Jerusalem, excessive work as well as army service had been his excuse for not visiting his father. The truth was that once Yoni's older brothers had left home, the strained atmosphere between himself and his father had not encouraged him to visit. While Yoni was growing up he had spent little time with his archeologist father who was usually involved in teaching, or his own projects. His injury provided him with a chance to visit the desert terrain he missed as well as an opportunity to visit his father and attempt to revive their relationship.

Yoni's arrival in Arad coincided with a spell of relentless scalding heat, followed by blustery sand storms, popularly known as a *sharev*. Though he found Jerusalem's vibe exciting, there had been times when he had longed for the solitude of the desert.

He considered himself fortunate to have grown up in Arad, on the edge of the Judean and Negev deserts, close to the Dead Sea, with biblical and archaeological significance. As a teenager, he'd often joined the tourists to view the ancient remains on the summit of the hill, *Tel Arad*, that stood over 40 metres, and above the plain.

Excavations in Arad revealed that two independent areas existed from two different periods in history: On the summit of the hill, were a number of fortresses and the only temple outside of Jerusalem built by the Israelites and Judeans.

However, Yoni was particularly interested in the excavations of a Canaanite city from the Bronze Age, located lower down on the southern slope of the hill. The well-planned city protected by thick walls and towers had been at the crossroads of major ancient trade routes. He had studied the way the Canaanites farmed, their use of metal for ploughing, their animals, and the wheat, barley and beans they once grew in the valley. The way in which ancient people lived intrigued Yoni. He had visited archaeological excavation sites in mountainous Northern Israel, called the Galilee, as well. Seeds discovered in the Galilee, revealed that the diet of people from around 10,000 years earlier, in the Neolithic Age, had consisted mainly of lentils, fava beans and chickpeas. He thought it incredible that people who had lived thousands of years ago had cultivated legumes, beans, and chickpeas, similar to the ones he cooked and served at the bistro.

Before Yoni had left for the city, he had enjoyed long walks in the desert. Now he longed for the desert's quiet freedom. As soon as the *sharev* passed, he set out as the rising sunlight shimmered across the mountains, canyons and craters. During his time away, he had almost forgotten the stark beauty of the vast landscape. With his injured arm in a sling, and the aid of a stick, he made his way across the rocky ground. There was always another rock formation or hauntingly beautiful mountain to admire in the distance.

He smiled to himself, remembering a morning desert walk after a sharev when he was seventeen. Then he had taken a path past the famous archaeological site in Arad, where he had been a volunteer sifting through rubble. He was younger then and unencumbered by a cast on his arm.

He must've covered at least fifteen kilometres, when he came across a heap of unusual looking stones exposed by the winds. His experience in volunteering at the archaeological dig told him that he may have found something of value. Wind storms frequently lifted layers of sand uncovering artifacts hidden below. Finding signs of earlier dwellers in the desert was a frequent occurrence. Carefully, he moved the stones and sand. Beneath were fragments of rubble, three large pieces of pottery, and two small ancient coins. A wad of earth dotted with seeds caught his attention as well. Carefully he wrapped the artefacts and piece of earth in his jumper and walked on.

When he returned home he placed his finds in a sealed box in the coolest part of the garage. It was a busy time of his life when his final school exams were facing him, followed by a long stint of training in the army. It wasn't surprising that he forgot about the box in the garage.

The heat of the sun returned Yoni to the present. He removed the warmer clothing he had started out with, and stuffed it into his backpack. He concluded that he was about a two hours walk from home, or possibly more. The artifacts he had found all those years ago were on his mind. He needed to return home to check if they were still where he had hidden them. How could he have been so irresponsible with his valuable find, he reproached himself. With his broken arm, the long, hot walk was more challenging than he had expected. He was forced to stop for sips of water and an occasional rest against a rock.

When he arrived home, he went directly to the garage. Within minutes he found the box he had hidden all those years ago. Relieved, he hurriedly opened it. All the items were intact and none the worse from their stay. At seventeen he had not appreciated the value of the artefacts, but he knew now that they could be valuable and important. That night he tossed and turned thinking about the box. When he woke, he decided that would seek his father's advice. As his father had assisted during the archeological dig at Arad, Yoni knew that he had chosen the best person to advise him.

'What an incredible discovery,' his father said excitedly, as he looked at the artefacts through a microscope. 'It's a pity you forgot about them, but that doesn't matter now,' he said, putting an arm around his son's shoulder. 'How amazing, the two bowls are only slightly cracked and the coins are in good condition. We must take them to the University of Jerusalem's Institute of Archaeology so that they can assess them. We'll drive there tomorrow.'

'What about that clod of earth with seeds? Do you think it's important?' Yoni asked.

'It might be the most important find of all. These seeds could even date back to very early times when ancient people relied on pulses for most of their meals. They planted pulses in the valleys from the dried seeds of previous crops, tended them until they were flourishing plants, and then had a supply to feed their people.'

'Who knows, they may even have made hummus.' Yoni laughed and slapped his thigh.

'Fava beans and chickpeas are as important a part of our diet now as they were for our biblical ancestors. Meat was a luxury in ancient times and pulses formed an important protein source. Each generation has passed on their knowledge to the next, and left their recipes,' his father said with a smile.

Yoni added, 'People might think earlier civilisations were backward or ignorant, but this shows how developed in their thinking they were. Today fewer people in the world would starve if they planted protein rich beans.'

'Indeed son. We must give thanks to our forefathers...and never forget them.'

Yoni and his father left for Jerusalem early the following morning. During the journey they talked more than they had for years. His father missed his mother, and much like Yoni, threw himself into work to fill the void in his life. Yoni had a lot to tell his father about the restaurant, and how successful it was becoming. The time passed so quickly that the journey seemed much shorter than they imagined.

They found the Institute of Archeology easily, but parking was another matter. At the university, Yoni showed one of the archeologists his find, and told her where the artifacts were discovered. She was only mildly interested in the coins and bowls.

'We have shelves full of these found in the desert, so you can keep them....but thank you for bringing them to our attention,' she said. She took a deep breath before continuing. 'This clod of earth with seeds attached is something very special...a spectacular find. We have only managed to excavate a few of these in the location you describe...so thank you...and you won't be getting it back.' She laughed, and placed the item in a box. 'We will try to date it and fully assess it. A very exciting find!'

As they walked back to the car, Yoni put his arm around his father's shoulder. 'Now that we've done our duty, it's time to enjoy ourselves. Our bistro is only a few blocks away. As you've not visited it yet, I want you to see it and try our food. Dan will be thrilled to see you, and will make us a delicious vegetarian lunch.'

His father smiled. 'A wonderful idea!'

The Mystical Lake

Lake Taupo is vast with a stretch of blue that disappears into the sky. There are so many stories about the lake's beauty and mystical qualities that I had to visit it when I went to New Zealand.

The magnificent lake lies in a crater of an inactive volcano with bubbling, thermal mud pools and icy spots. I tried to swim in it, but gave up. The water felt heavy and had a strange mineral smell.

One afternoon, I took a cruise on a replica of an old steamboat. Sailing with the breeze on the water was a welcome escape from the hot day. The passengers were a mix of people, tourists like myself.

The boat moved slowly over the smooth water.

'The Maoris are a Polynesian people who arrived here between 1150 and 1350,' the guide said.

The motion of the boat relaxed me as his voice droned on with historical facts about the volcano that had created the lake.

The boat sidled up to tall rocks covered in Maori carvings. On the nearest rock, an enormous warlike mask was heavily carved, and on the surrounding rocks were animals from Maori legends. The mask both frightened and repulsed me. I interpreted it as a "keep out" sign to all strangers. I felt sure that the masked face guarded not only the lake, but the mountain behind it as well.

'Strange things can happen on these waters,' the guide said without further explanation.

A few sceptical murmurs came from the passengers.

'You don't believe me?' the guide muttered with a shrug and stared out towards the horizon for several minutes before speaking again. 'I'll tell you what happened to me about ten years ago, and you can judge for yourselves.'

I sat up and waited.

'I was going through a terrible time, then,' he said, as he began his story. 'I had split up with my wife and was living alone. I was so shaken up that I couldn't even sail my boat. I suppose I got used to being alone after a time. One afternoon, I felt like sailing again. As the sun dipped down, I headed for home. It was then that I saw it in the distance, a canoe manned by Maori warriors moving like a fast machine. Then, as they came from nowhere, they disappeared.'

A roar of comments came from the people around me. At the time I wondered why he was telling us this story and if he told the same one to every load of passengers he ferried around the lake.

'Please, let me finish the story. It's a special one...I only tell it occasionally.'

I nodded to myself cynically.

He glanced at us, straightened his shoulders and continued. 'The word goes that many years ago a Maori chief saw a canoe on the lake just before a massive volcano blew its top, destroying villages in this area. People around here say he thought it was a sign of coming disaster...and he was right.' He lit a cigarette and took a draw. 'I knew the story, so you must know how scared I was of what I'd seen that day. I sailed back to the harbour in a hurry to ask if anyone else had seen the canoe. But none of the sailors had seen it.'

He had a drink of water and continued his story. 'I put my vision of the canoe down to tiredness or imagination, and forgot about it until one Sunday about six months later. The day was stormy. I was trying to stay afloat in churning waters near the deepest part of the lake when I saw the canoe again. This time it was closer and the carved red wood and all the oarsmen were clear. There must've been a dozen men with bare chests wearing grass skirts. Their bodies and faces were covered with tattoos. In spite of the enormous waves that day, they rowed together and swept through that water like one man. The men rode towards the shore, and then onto the sand of the lake beach. They climbed out, and their women folk and children ran to greet them. They hugged and raced up the beach together. Then the pictured faded. The beach was empty. '

'Weird,' a man behind me said.

'So what did you make of it?' I called out to the guide. He held up his hand again to stop me and the others questioning him.

'All I can say is that seeing them made a change to my life,' he said, as he steered the steamship into its berth.

I shook my head, puzzled by the unsatisfactory ending to his story. Our trip was over and a queue waited for the next tour. We filed off the boat while he busied himself with the new group of passengers.

After my stay at Taupo I returned to Auckland. When I arrived home, I found that my girlfriend had moved out of the house we had shared. I can't say I was surprised, as we hadn't been getting along for months. Being alone in the house unsettled me. I flung myself into work. Soon I was almost as tired as I had been before the holiday. In spite of my efforts, I missed out on a promotion to someone with better qualifications. The disappointment knocked me about.

Weeks later, I saw a poster in the city mall advertising Maori singing and dancing. The image of the masked head guarding the watery wall came back to me as clearly as the day I had seen it. That night, over a cold beer or two, I thought about the guide's story. What it had meant to the guide wasn't important, nor whether it was true or not. That it was back in my thoughts, told me that it had to be important to me. Days later, the story's special meaning, hit me. I was unsettled and feeling alone. My job wasn't satisfying, and I had cut myself off from people close to me - my parents, relatives, old school friends and work mates. I had chosen to ignore the warning signs, the nervous roar inside me. I needed to be one of a team rowing with others and welcomed home. At last, I understood. I didn't feel that I belonged. That was it!

Though it's not easy, I'm trying my best. I've taken the plunge. I'm looking for a new job. There are a few interviews for jobs coming up this week. I've contacted one or two old friends and I'll be having lunch with Mum and Dad this Sunday. As long as I take it slowly, I'll sort myself out.

An Important Visit

It was the Sabbath, the holiest day of the week, and Leah was late for synagogue. She took a deep breath before she climbed the stairs to the women's gallery. She hesitated, wondering if she had worn the right outfit, and if it made her look fat. Wherever she went she was self-conscious about her weight.

The service had already begun. Amongst the women's faces she recognised many and greeted them. She smiled, nodded and puzzled over the names of others. Trying her best not to disturb the women around her, she made her way to her seat. During a lengthy prayer, she looked around at the other worshippers. Some she knew were struggling with illness, personal sadness, financial woes, or family problems. An old, arthritic woman, a survivor of the Holocaust sitting next to her, struggled to turn the pages of her prayer book. What was important is that she had survived and was there. A grey haired woman sitting in front of her, usually immaculately dressed was in black, her hair unkempt. She was battling to stem her tears. But they were all there, still together.

Leah glanced at all the worshipers around her, pondering on how as a people they had survived, and how their beliefs and rituals had remained intact. The interior of synagogues had hardly changed over the centuries of worship. The prayers were not much altered either. She cast her mind back to the many situations in history that could easily have wiped them out, yet they were thriving while many other civilizations and religions had come and gone.

The mumble of prayer rose, as the cantor intoned the ancient chants. A quiet calm pervaded her. The loose fragments of her being came together, made her feel whole again. She felt connected to all that had gone before, and what was spiritual for her now. As always, when she attended synagogue, she thought of her parents, her extended family, and friends who had all passed on. They were only memories now, and missing them was part of her life.

A soft voice whispered. It was Len, who had died a few years earlier. 'Tell her…please. …that she's the love of my life.'

Then a friend's ninety year old mother, still elegant in the blue outfit Leah had liked best, appeared in a shimmer, smiled her lovely smile, and then disappeared.

Where were her parents, she wondered. 'If only they would visit.'

After the service, she and her family ate the lunch she had prepared. They talked, sharing the week's events and relaxed, enjoying the Sabbath. She had time to ponder on the voice she had heard, and the vision of her friend's mother. Nothing like that had happened to her before, though she was an intuitive person. After some thought, she dismissed the idea that her visitors were imaginary, or that there was something wrong with her brain. The messages were meaningful and had come at a time when she was self-absorbed. Her weight and the clothes she wore were irrelevant. There were so many friends and others in her community to whom she could offer a listening ear, or support in their difficulties. Some were missing from the service due to ill health.

She would contact her two friends and deliver the messages she had received. Then she would make enquiries about joining the group of volunteers who visited sick members, or helped in other ways. Perhaps she could visit people who had lost loved ones, and some others in the community, and help where she could. She reflected that mutual support was one of the reasons that the small community was still vital and functioning.

Acknowledgements

I would like to thank my husband Hymie for his love and support over the two years I spent in compiling my stories, as well the ideas and suggestions he contributed. Special thanks go members of my writing group, The Avenue Writer's Collective, for their constant encouragement and constructive editing.

The help from Estelle, Topsy, Gita and others who read drafts of the book, and assisted with proofreading was invaluable. All my friends who listened patiently to my ideas about stories deserve my thanks too.

My thanks and gratitude goes to Sylvie Blair for her interest in this project, all her work in turning my manuscript into this book, and her attention to detail.

As always, all errors are my own.

www.ingramcontent.com/pod-product-compliance
Lightning Source LLC
Chambersburg PA
CBHW060251100426
42742CB00011B/1707